The Bio-Mystical Womb Journal

A Guided Journey Towards Your Bio-Mystical Womb Wellness

By

Jessica Huckabay

Reviews

"This book is a deep dive into the essential art of self-reflection. There is not enough of it in the world! The base of all healing, as inscribed above the Temple doors in Delphi "know thyself, and forgive". Jessica weaves through the stages of life, development, elements, to help find the jewels of self-discovery to assist in your womb journey. The food and herbs plus the resourceful links ensure you will have a wealth of connections, information and choices to be healed and healthy. The poems and personal quotes help weave and inspire throughput. A treasure trove of gems. I know this journal is going to help many women. Blessed be" Angie Twydall, Womb Healer and training facilitator, founder of the Sanctuary of Sophia

"This book soars past the non-fiction wellness genre and reads like a piece of art and a spiritual journey. Poetry, journaling, practices, and guidance…I feel this book is not filling my head with facts but moving through my body, my womb's center.

Huckabay addresses the sexism and domination culture that keeps us from caring for our wombs. It is trauma-informed focused on our care, giving us tools to navigate the complexities of diving into our wombs and our ancestors that gave us life through their wombs. Huckabay invites us to guide ourselves on our own journey through this book and it feels nurturing and empowering to read it.

As a trans person, I feel touched and grateful that Huckabay sought to include us so thoughtfully. I hope my LGBTQ+ community can benefit from this work. We need more books that dive into the brave world of getting back in touch with our bodies and our creativity that also consider us thoughtfully.

This book leaves space not just for wellness, but for wholeness." Dylan Wilder Quinn, TransIntimate

"The Bio-Mystical Womb Journal creates a beautiful space between sharing and asking in order to listen. I'm used to 'healing paths' being about set structures and one-way practices. It is so refreshing to have the freedoms of creativity celebrated as a resource rather than a hinderance to any set, one-way methodology. Jessica honors her values to support others to find and hear guidance that is their own, not anyone else's." Evie Grifiths, Visionary Poet

"If you are ready to do The Work, release the past, and create ancestral healing... then this book is for you. Jessica Huckabay's Journal Journey gives you a capability that most do not. Most authors will guide you in a certain direction. Jessica allows you to find your own direction, your own answers, and your own guidance from within. With a little facilitation and Womb Shamanic questions, Jessica even recommends to use this book in a non-linear fashion for purposes of learning your automatic intuitive womb wisdom and watching how the question, "randomly" picked, will be perfect for where you are in life. You trusted your intuition enough to look at this book and read this specific review. Trust your intuition once again by buying this book and committing to your womb practice by sitting down, going in, and answering these questions. See you in Mother Earths collective womb sanctuary! In this life or the next." - Jaslin Varzideh, Co-Founder of Red Tent Goddess

"An engaging and powerful guide for your womb wisdom journey. Jessica is knowledgeable and supportive with her beautiful words. Whether you are only beginning or wish to strengthen your womb wisdom connection this journal will be useful and nourishing. Do it for you, your ancestors and the generations to come." Crystal Waters of Making Mundane Magical

"A deep dive with little jewels along the way as you rediscover and tread through your unique journey." Arishna Ramnath, philanthropist and seeker

"If you are looking for a book that will deepen the connection with ancestral wombs, your womb and the wombs that come through you, this is the book for you. The Bio-Mystical Womb Journal has allowed me to continue and intensify my ancestral healing journey. It has given me the necessary tools to support my daughters current and future womb journeys as well as a book to continue the work that I've started." Nneka J. Hall

"This book in the style of a journal is alive with inspirational questions, prompts and poetic musings; the aim of which is to stir your deepest inner knowing. Filled with the author's own creative womb wisdom your imagination and intuition are activated, enabling you to connect to your own unique feminine wisdom. Its pages provide a place for you to record and discover your own depth of meaning as you delve into the poignant prompts. It's a comprehensive map for your own personal development. Jessica has put together this book as a remembrance into the truth of who you are, deep from the wisdom of the body.

This book also holds within it nourishing wisdom gleaned from participants that have taken part in Jessica's online programs. Each nugget of knowing the women have shared lets you know you are connected to a collective of ancient linages of womb wisdom. This book is a true guide that also includes practical information on herbal wisdom, suggested practices and where to seek professional support. It will open locked doors into the deepest central parts of you, right at the core of your own being." Coco Oya Cienna-Rey

"Wow, wow, wow. This is a journal for those ready to truly do the work of healing and sitting in their sacred seat. As a Holistic Health Practitioner that specializes in womb wellness, I can foresee not only recommending but requiring this journal for every client I work with. This journal takes us all, experienced and novice, on a deep dive into our inner divine consciousness awakening the power to hear our true inner voice, our womb's voice. I love that it's a journal that can be revisited time and time again throughout this lifetime. May everyone that uses this medicine be blessed as I have been. Tua Neter" Practitioner Michelle, Founder of Soulfully Healthy Living and co-founder of D&D Life Farms

"I recognized many of the questions from the journal that were so helpful during the 13 Months Bio-Mystical Womb Apprenticeship. I found the poems so inviting to connect to my own womb wisdom and develop my inner listening and receiving answers in the form of images and metaphors. I loved the re-weaving in stages of ancestors, conception, birth, enchantress...Including the elements rounded it off as well. Overall, such a deep space to deeply dive into the ocean of our own womb and so healing, too." Erika Maizi, Author, Soul based Coach, Visionary Artist and Founder of the Wyrding Way

"This is a very thought provoking, and truly spiritually nourishing book for women seeking to connect to the voice of their wombs. Jessica's eloquent words, and soothing poetic style of writing really brings emotional awareness to the hidden voice within the depths of our wombs. I undoubtedly recommend this journal to any woman that is desiring to connect more deeply with their intuition, ancestral patterns, and voice of her womb. You will come away more empowered to live your truth, and ready to offer your innate Divine gifts to the world. Get your journal today, no hesitations, just do it!" Oshun, Leading Women's Holistic Health Practitioner, Menstrual Cycle Coach, Womb Priestess, and Feminine Transformation Leader

"I am so thrilled to have gotten the gift of reading this and writing a review. The intro I can feel the nurturing empowering intent. This drew me in closer. Reading the intro was a welcoming home, an invitation. I feel this is such a gift to the reader. The questions, I love how they embrace and hold feminine power with grace and wisdom. I love the inclusivity; we all hold womb space. For me personally this was a very healing section. I love the depth of each question. The questions bring gentle, comforting questions, so the reader can find their own wisdom within. I love the gentle, yet empowering questions that lead the reader to inner wisdom.

The poem (TO SEE THE PLACES I SEE) brings spirit, DNA, soul of our womb spaces to the healing of our world. We all belong. We are holy and sacred. (GRANDMOTHERS, HONEY, COCOON) Wow!! Nourishing and holy. Each poem touches parts of the other and brings the reader back to our womb wisdom. This is a needed piece of work. I see a recent change in womb wisdom coming more open into the world. I feel this journal is as an important part of that evolution." Raymora Thomas, Writer

"This is really a valuable book and practice to integrate on any woman's journey! Your approach is the first one that really got my attention in this field of womb centering and healing. It is such a different approach, because you walk your talk by following the guidance of the womb and give us the same opportunity while working with the journal.

I am new in this practice of womb listening but I feel the calling. I really do. It started with your book. I had a few sessions of connecting with the womb and I can't say that I have reached the stage where I 'hear' the guidance but I felt a few things. I feel a connection with something deep inside me, a whole universe, not just about me but about something larger and feminine in a universal sense, not just personal.

It helped me to relax in a more profound way, to quiet the noise in my mind and emotional storms just by placing my hands on my womb and breathing. It brings me back into my body. I am very aware of my body but the womb centering brings me even closer. There is a sense of unity between the upper and the lower part of my body as in superior-inferior type of energies. Usually I feel a separation between them but this practice brings acceptance and a feeling of integration of the creative, sexual energy.

An interesting insight during the last session was the feeling that "this is where my sky begins", in the womb. It is quite surprising and I am looking forward to discover more about my sky because I didn't expect to find it there.

I work with the womb on a daily basis since I teach oriental dance and one of the main styles of the Egyptian Dance is Baladi. Baladi starts in the womb and it is a direct, raw exploration of the creative energy. It is about listening, deep listening and improvising by following what the womb and the music are saying. It is both sensual and earthy, internalized but creative. But I still feel I have a lot to discover inside or outside the dance by listening to the womb. And I am sure that my practice will help me and my students to improve not just in dance but also in our journey to be more feminine, alive, connected and wise. Thank you so much for bringing this into the world and sharing it with us. For me it's just a beginning but I'll follow the calling." Cerasela Magdalena, Oriental Dance teacher

"The Bio-Mystical Womb Journal is a bio-mystical initiation. The title alone starts to activate a connection to your womb wherever you are on your own womb journey and it has enhanced my connection to my own womb. This journal is a beautiful, unique experience that surpasses the boundaries of most books as it engages you to dive into your womb wisdom right from the start with a simple practice to begin connecting to your womb. It assumes you can do this and after a brief inspiring context setting you start. I was very surprised that I could access my womb in this particular journaling way. I was very inspired by Jessica's own poems and womb writings- they are beautiful and make me want to dive in more to develop this ability to write from my womb. The experience is deep and grounding and brings me home deeper to myself. I love the simplicity and the depth of this journal." Michelle White Hart, Womb Power: Movement & Meditation Journey

"This book is grounding. Jessica takes us on a journey through the seasons of our womb lives providing clarity, understanding and honesty with compassion and support. Through this book, she also teaches, highlighting various subjects once considered taboo, removing stigma or shame replace with love, embrace and support. Thank you for your selfless work!" Tracy Shearer, Holistic Health Practitioner & Wellness Coach, Flourish With Tracy

This book is dedicated to all of the supportive influences that have converged to allow me to write this book. My husband Geoffrey Huckabay, my mother Teresa Todd-Ingram, the case study apprentices in the Bio-Mystical Womb Apprenticeship program, and all of my previous and current mentors, the list of which is too long to include here. It is also dedicated to non-human supporters like the members of the garden community, the forest community, the waters of the rivers, lakes, underground water ways, ocean, and waters falling from the sky, the air, the fire, and Mother Earth, without which none of us would be here. It is also dedicated to the Wisdom Ancestors who have extracted spiritual nourishment from their lifetimes to deliver as medicine to me and all who are available to receive it. Thank you all for teaching me how we can all come together in our unique ways and be in community despite what might get in our way.

Table of Contents

Introduction

Congratulations on responding to the inner nudge you felt when you saw this book to take the step to nurture your womb wellness by purchasing it and opening to this page.

The intention of this book is to provide a structure and gentle guidance for you to explore your Bio-Mystical Womb Wisdom and let it guide your personal and collective Womb Wellness journey. This book includes some instructional and inspirational materials, but it is mostly a journal for you to inquire inwards, connect with your inner guidance, and fill the pages with your own unique version of this wisdom.

In my experience, most of our womb imbalances and ailments arise from the mass hypnosis that has been teaching us and our ancestors for many generations to prioritize external authority and intellectual knowledge about what is important in our lives. As these sources of authority and knowledge have been heavily shaped by the influence of domination-based models of relationship, womb wellness has landed time and again at the bottom of the priority list. In fact, our wombs have largely been relegated to the list of 'natural resources' to be exploited.

And when our wombs have cried out in pain at this treatment, we have been told that this is 'normal'. Which is true. It is normal to cry out in pain when we are exploited for the benefit of others and to the detriment of ourselves.

I have been blessed with many mentors who have kept ancient traditions of womb reverence alive or done the work of reclaiming these traditions despite the mass hypnosis described above. One of the fundamental teachings of these traditions that is deeply revolutionary on both personal and collective levels is that of partnership instead of domination in our relationships. Partnership requires us to see all parties in a relationship as valid contributors to any decision-making process. This requires we listen to each other, especially to those who have typically been ignored and over-ridden within the domination model. This means listening to our bodies instead of dominating them, and especially our wombs and menstrual cycles, for the valuable feedback and information they are giving us about how our lifestyle choices are affecting our well-being.

At some point on my journey of implementing this wisdom, I realized that my womb was a source of powerful wisdom that has been recognized in many traditions around the world. Modern science is only recently beginning to understand this and start to emerge from the deeply destructive suppression of this wisdom. As we collectively come up for air, many womb reverence practitioners are discovering the practice of listening to their own womb wisdom and letting it guide their lives, to great regenerative effect.

This book is designed to help you discover and/or deepen this practice of womb listening for yourself. This might be quite different than other books that you may have read in an attempt to learn something new. Most non-fiction books are filled with loads of information and instructions about how to learn and implement the teachings the authors are writing about.

I had plans to write this book in that way. But at a certain point I realized that it would never be finished. There was an infinite amount of information and instructions that could be written about reclaiming our womb wisdom and my womb wisdom kept telling me that I needed to publish this book sooner than that.

After much reflection and deep feeling, it became clear that I had already finished writing the book. I had written a set of questionnaires to accompany the Bio-Mystical Womb Apprenticeship program that I designed around the teachings I planned to eventually share in this book. They contained questions that had nourished my womb wellness journey as well as that of the participants in the apprenticeship. Several of the participants had submitted their responses to the questions as case study participants with the agreement that I could include their writings in this book to inspire others who were embarking on the journey by reading it. And much of my writings intended to be included in this book have been inspired by the questions as well.

So even though I could write this book to highlight my expertise, thereby fortifying the mass hypnosis that says that the knowledge and authority you need is somewhere outside of you, I have chosen instead to listen to my own womb wisdom and write this book as a guide for you to connect with your inner knowledge.

My hope is that you will use this book as an interactive tool to nurture your own partnership with your womb wisdom and let it guide you to greater and greater well-being. The journaling prompts included in this book will often offer suggestions of practices you can start with to connect more deeply with your womb wisdom. There will also be snippets of writings I or some of the case study apprentices have done in response to the questions to inspire and motivate you to keep writing. Soon we will have written a book together in partnership and community. My womb wisdom couldn't be happier about this.

The questions in this book are organized around the timeline of our lifecycles, guiding us to revisit all the ways we have experienced womb wisdom, from our parental womb space all the way through to the death portal and our inevitable return to the Cosmic Womb. You are welcome to write your way through this journal in a linear fashion, following this timeline. However, I will say that this is not how my womb wisdom journey occurred. Over the years of reclaiming the wisdom from all the womb initiations that were neglected or missed throughout my life, I have jumped around on the timeline, revisiting moments of import in a very non-linear fashion, depending on what was happening in my life that brought my awareness to a particular developmental phase or experience that left me in need of a certain skill or quality in the current circumstance.

There seems to be an intrinsic intelligence at play guiding my journey of reclamation based on what is needed at any given moment. To honor this intelligence in you, I invite you to explore a non-linear approach to working with this book, perhaps by opening it at random to journal from time to time or thumbing through the pages to find a journaling question that feels relevant to your current inner landscape. Better yet, drop into a womb listening inquiry and ask your own womb wisdom which journaling questions to write about today.

A note on gender and the womb:

We were all born from a womb. We all have reproductive physiology that originated from the same cluster of cells. We all have energetic centers associated with our connection to our soul and creativity in the same area of our body. We can all connect with a womb space or womb center in similar ways. Some of us have physical wombs and others do not, but this does not determine our gender biology or identity. We all have a womb journey anyways.

To nurture every gender who might feel called to explore their womb center with the support of this book, I have chosen to use gender neutral terms when at all possible. This book does use gendered terms at times like Goddess, Mama, Mermaid, specifically when I (or other writing contributors) am (are) describing my (their) own experiences through poetry, storytelling, and reviews. I invite your creativity into this work and to alter the words so that they affirm your own journey.

In this process I have discovered that this also nurtures the full spectrum of family configurations folks may have experienced growing up, which feels lovely too, as my womb wisdom seems to guide me towards ever greater care for as many folks as possible.

If you do feel a deep connection between your gender and womb, whether a physical or spiritual womb, I honor that and invite you to nurture that connection, while also opening to the idea that other people may have a different relationship to their gender and womb.

Please take a moment to place your hands on your wombs space, take some deep breaths, and ask your womb wisdom for any insights you might have about the topics above. Write out your reflections here:

A Note on Gender Dysphoria and Euphoria around bellies and wombs

The womb and belly can be a source of dysphoria and trauma for some trans and gender expansive people, and of distress and trauma for cisgender people as well. I invite you to move at your own pace with this work, to use this work as a source of resilience-building and healing for any dysphoria or distress that may come up.

If you experience dysphoria or distress around your womb and belly, I invite you to take breaks at times to use a resilience practice of grounding yourself into parts of your body that you feel euphoria around, or a lack of distress or gender dysphoria...parts of your body that you are enjoying in this moment, such as your voice, your hair, the tip of your nose, your ankle bone, your pinky toe, your lungs, or your heart....any part of your body you feel in relationship with. Take a few breaths here, and notice your relationship with this part of your body. Ground in your joy, contentment, connection with this part of your body. Use this tool as needed throughout this book.

Please take a few moments now to write about how you might care for any dysphoria and/or euphoria you may encounter as you explore connecting with your womb space and belly in your own way. Do any of the suggestions here sound nurturing and supportive? Is there any wisdom and/or insight arising for you from your past experiences or intuition that you could make a note of here to come back to remind yourself as needed?

Notes on intuitive herbalism and when to seek professional support:

Throughout this journal, you will be invited to connect intuitively with plants and explore inner guidance around how they might support you. Plants have evolved with humanity, and many have deeply nourishing and beneficial qualities. Many, however, are quite toxic or can be in certain circumstances. I highly recommend that you research any plant you connect with intuitively before ingesting it. Your intuitive connection may be symbolic or metaphorical and we do not need to ingest plants to receive their benefit.

I also encourage you to seek out the support of professional herbalists if you are experiencing difficult symptoms, especially around your menstrual cycle, and especially if your symptoms have stumped the medical professionals you have consulted. Your intuitive connections with plants will be a lovely supplement to the support of a trained herbalist in creating an herbal womb wellness plan. Naturopathic doctors, Functional Medicine Doctors, Chinese Medicine practitioners and Ayurvedic doctors can all offer holistic support as well.

The second part of this book includes self-assessment questions and more detailed suggestions about when to seek professional support, so if you are having intense symptoms, you might want to jump ahead to that portion of the book.

You can also take a moment now to place your hands on your womb space and listen to the intensity of the messages your womb is giving you through your symptoms. Feel the intensity of the emotions you have around your symptoms. Ask your inner wisdom for guidance about how important it is to get professional support to bring your systems back into balance. Write out any insights you receive on this and any strategies you can implement to prioritize your womb wellness by finding practitioners to support you.

Take another moment to connect with your inner wisdom and reflect on what feelings or circumstances might be stopping you from seeking out and getting the professional care that you need for your womb wellness. Write out your reflections here and any solutions or strategies you could implement to overcome these obstacles and get the care you need.

PART I: Bio-Mystical Womb Early Life Cycle Initiation Journey

In this part we will begin with practices and reflections about the early phases of our womb life cycle journey. This includes the time before our conception when our spirit may have consulted with ancestors and other allies and guides about our purpose in this life. It also includes our conception, gestation, and birth processes as well as our early childhood and coming of age.

The questions in this part (and in all the parts really) may bring up emotions and memories that have been buried as they weren't safe to feel at the time they originated. I invite you to take some time to reflect on how you might nurture and support yourself on this journey of deep inner listening and write out some strategies in response to these initial questions below.

I suggest starting with a womb listening practice of placing your hands on your belly, taking at least 5 deep nourishing, relaxing breaths, letting out sighing and/or yawning sounds on the exhale, stretching and wiggling to relax more if that feels good to you, and then bringing your awareness to your womb space, just below your navel and back towards your spine. Imagine a golden seed of light in your womb space that sprouts a root down through your pelvic floor that reaches all the way to the surface of Mother Earth. Give your love and gratitude to Mother Earth with another exhale down through your root and then inhale her vital energy and wisdom into your womb. Let this vital energy and wisdom create an imaginary womb sanctuary with a wise womb membrane that surrounds you and only allows in beneficial energies. Imagine how your womb sanctuary might be furnished and decorated to nourish and support you. Then open your eyes and write out some answers from your womb wisdom to these questions:

- How does it feel to connect with your womb space as a source of wisdom and guidance?

- How might you enlist the support of your loved ones, friends, and professional support team while you embark on this journey?

- How might you set up a sacred space for your journey? What comforts, beauties, and pleasures might you gather and arrange to support yourself?

- How might you organize your time to prioritize this journey?

- Is there anyone you might like to invite to join you on this journey? How will you hold each other accountable to the commitment you are making to embark on this journey together?

- How do you plan to care for yourself if difficult material comes up for you along this journey? What strategies work well for you if you feel overwhelmed with emotions or physically unwell?

- Who can you call upon for support with intense emotional processes or physical symptoms?

- How do you know when you need to call upon your support people or recovery strategies? What are some signs you have noticed in the past that you need to regroup and recover?

- How do you know when you have returned to a place of stability and readiness to explore more? What signs of readiness and stability do you notice when you feel rested and resourced?

Chapter One:

Pre-conception, Conception, Gestation, and Birth

You are invited to gather your comforts, beauties, and pleasures and settle in for some womb listening time. Set up your space as guided by your womb wisdom in the Part One Intro.

I suggest starting with a womb listening practice of placing your hands on your belly, taking at least 5 deep nourishing, relaxing breaths, letting out sighing and/or yawning sounds on the exhale, stretching and wiggling to relax more if that feels good to you, and then bringing your awareness to your womb space. Imagine a golden seed of light in your womb space that sprouts a root down through your pelvic floor that reaches all the way to the surface of Earth. Give your love and gratitude to Earth with another exhale down through your root and then inhale her vital energy and wisdom into your womb. Let this vital energy and wisdom create an imaginary womb sanctuary with a wise womb membrane that surrounds you and only allows in beneficial energies. Imagine how your womb sanctuary might be furnished and decorated to nourish and support you. Then open your eyes and write out some answers from your womb wisdom to these questions:

Pre-conception and Conception

What do you know about your ancestral heritage? What questions do you have? How might you research this information and find out more?

Imagine that you have an ancient ancestor, or perhaps more than one, who is well of spirit and well of womb, from back before all of the womb wounding societal structures came to be. What does this ancestor look like? Feel like?

The Places I am From

By Jessica Huckabay

To see the places I am from

Stretches the senses back farther than my birth

Back into the warm waters where I was formed

Back into the waiting seed carried inside her

Carried inside my Grandmother

Who was carried inside her mother

Stretching back like a house of mirrors

Smaller and smaller images of me

In the infinite dreams and prayers

Of my ancestors

I am from tear moistened hands

Crocheting in the rocking chair

A rhythmic longing for the lost jungle

I am from plague-stricken evacuations to the mountains

Cooler weather offering solace, health, and financial ruin

Fueling transatlantic boat journeys in search of an elusive livelihood

Chasing a stolen promise

Leaving all of true value behind

I am from people owned by the land

Owned by their bodies

Owned by nature

Torn from their belonging

By the wounded hands of greed

I am from those wounded hands

Bathing their offspring

In blood

Twisting the god of love

Into the god of war

The god of slavery

Claiming permission to decide who has a soul and who does not

I am from hands held up

Flat to the face of this war god

Voices saying no

Feet walking away from safety and security

Hearts longing for

Remembering the holy source of love

In our bellies

In the rivers

In the mountains

In the trees

In the sky

In the smell of roses

Recognizing the soul

In all things

I am from all things

Praying for the recognition of their soul

I am from Mother Earth

Deciding

Enough is enough

Gasping awake

From dark dreams of what could be possible

If she doesn't start finding the feet

Of the two-leggeds ready

To hear her voice

Feel her love

Recognize her soul once more

How does this poem inspire you?

Write out a conversation with your ancient wisdom ancestor asking them any questions you might have about your soul purpose and writing out what you imagine their answers might be.

Grandmother's Honey Cocoon

By Jessica Huckabay

I stand at the center of a rainbow mandala

Glowing orbs of light surround me

Floating in concentric circles

I hear voices echoing from these orbs

Some sing sweetly

Of divine union

Some cry out and grown with the weight of disconnection and despair

Their colors are muted

Covered with sticky charred oil

Their center light dimmed by longing

They hang low and heavy

When they notice my attention they try to come close

Get inside my body

Live again through me

My light a beacon

Grandmother welcomes them at the edges of my membrane

Scoops them into a great golden cocoon

Where they can steep for as many thousands of years as needed

In the golden honey of divine motherly love

This honey slowly dissolves their crusty burnt edges

Softens and lightens their burdens

Waves of forgiveness pulse through this cocoon

Their patterns of pain slowly change shape

Shedding layers of illusion

Until the wisdom is revealed

As their spiritual hearts lighten

Their inner light brightens

They float closer to the top of the cocoon

As their wisdom ripens, portals open for them to be born

They become wisdom ancestors

Well of spirit

No longer hungry to repeat their pain patterns

Having digested them fully

They can now offer nourishment to others

As I digest these pain patterns in my own body

I send the nourishment that overflows inside of me

Into this golden cocoon

This is not a burden for me

As I receive so abundantly from Grandmother

And all of the wisdom ancestors

We all generate our own light

Our own living honey nectar

We return any threads of stolen nourishment to its rightful owners

We contribute to the waves of divine motherly love

Washing over the ones still in the cocoon

Grandmother places her hand on my shoulder

She gazes out over this mandala of healing with me

She smiles and nods

"It is well" she says

And I agree

"But what if there is a healing needed that feels too grave for me? There are so many wounded spirits...:" I ask her.

"I will help you. I have been doing this for much longer than you can imagine. I will   show you the way."

I sigh with relief and rest back into her warm, wrinkled hand

The pain in my shoulder melts under its warmth

And I am lost in our unified pulse of life

How does this poem inspire you?

Imagine how your ancient wisdom ancestor might support you with any healing processes you need to do around any ancestral womb wounding you carry in your womb space. Write out any guidance or assistance you imagine this ancient wisdom ancestor might have for you.

If you were to create a space in your womb healing sanctuary to honor this ancient wisdom ancestor, what would they have you place in that space as offerings and reminders of their presence and support for you?

Grandmother

By Jessica Huckabay

Grandmother brings feathers and wings into the room and offers her husky voice into the air. She sings the rhythms of transformation, the pulse of smoke. Her arm flies through the air, feeling the movements of energy in the subtle inflections of her feathers and the heartbeat of the person lying there learning how to breath again.

Grandmother has held this ceremony of healing uncountable times. They flow together. It is all one ceremony. Each person that finds themself in her presence is the same person. We all need the same ceremony. The ceremony to remember the breath, to reignite the inner fire. The ceremony to clear the inner rivers of dams and debris. The ceremony to re-center the womb, reconnect to the blood. The ceremony of stones, of bones, of becoming earth again, feeling our feet on the ground. The ceremony of returning to life, returning to love.

Grandmother feels time like a piercing light that contains all things at once. The people flash in and out before her, in need of her eternal ceremony. The planets turn, flourish, ail, die, and are reborn as her feathers caress space. The sun grows hotter and colder, stars expand and disappear, people, animals, civilizations all pulsing in and out of existence.

I thought Grandmother was visiting me. But it turns out sometimes an opening happens and I am with her. I thought she was doing the ceremony for me and whomever I was with, but she is just eternally being Grandmother, in ceremony, loving life into existence.

Grandmother knows when I am there with her. She knows what I know and don't know. She knows her feather dance, her voice seems to be just what we need right now. She knows that we don't know that that is always true. But now we know because she just smiled that smile that spreads this type of knowing through the air, she just sang that song that places insight and wisdom in our wombs without words. She just followed that air current with the tip of her feather that opened the veils of illusion just enough for me and you to smell her incense for a moment and recognize the roses in our garden, the rosemary in our potatoes, the blood of our wombs in that aroma.

As soon as we begin to awaken to her eternal presence inside of us, the feather slips away from that opening, the veils shimmer shut, and we forget enough to keep us hungry. Hungry enough to go looking for Grandmother. Hungry enough to find her.

How does this writing inspire you?

How might you and your ancient wisdom ancestor prepare the womb sanctuary to facilitate healing in your relationships with ancestors that feel difficult to connect with? What comforts, beauties and pleasures might you add to the space? What healing technologies might you set up?

Forgiveness

By Jessica Huckabay

Forgiveness

Is a waterfall it turns out

One I have visited many times in my imagination

It flows into gently tiered crystalline pools

Extending into a river

And all the way to the sea

I have dreamt about this same river my whole life

I always know how to get there in my dreams

Anywhere I have lived in waking life

Has an access point to this river in my dreams

In waking life I find myself looking for it

Knowing it is there

But only arriving again in dreams

Where we float and swim downstream together

Smiling and laughing

At the coolness

The wisdom

The softness of the water

That infuses happiness into us

In waking dreams I have visited the source

This waterfall

Where the Goddess herself seems to be

Delivering her clear elixir of forgiveness

But the kind that simply erases all harm with its flow

Not to the point of forgetting

But infusing all hurts with wisdom

I find gifts at the bottom of this clear pool

Absorb them into my dream body

I bring bowls of rage to the edge of this pool

Bowls of fire, almost too hot to touch

Carried in slings

On yolks over my shoulders

I ask this waterfall to put out these flames

Soothe these burns

I am shown a circle of bowls in a cave under the waterfall

My fires are too hot to be extinguished by these gentle waters

Or the mist

As I enter the cave

To meet Grandmother

Who invites me to sit inside the circle

I must lower my yolk

Placing my still flaming bowls

In the empty spots in the circle

And join her next to the fire in the ground

I see how our glowing bowls light up the darkness

Revealing pathways into the mountain

I can hear the sounds of activity

People, animals, wind, water, and fire

Dancing in the tunnels

Echoing with life

"Why do you want to put out these flames?"

Grandmother asks me

"They have burned me so many times. I am hot, irritated,

 I cannot speak without shouting

My fluids are drying up

My tissues are inflamed" I reply

"Ahhh, you have forgotten to dance.

You have been too busy to visit the river."

"You must remember to sing the song of water

And breath with the wind

This will balance out these flames

And return them to their nourishing usefulness

Allowing you to forgive yourself

And anyone else who has experienced causing harm to others"

Grandmother tells me as she begins to beat her drum

She sings the song of the river

To remind me

I feel her drum and her voice moving my body

I am dancing around the center fire

Stepping around and through the outer circle of fires

Offerings that so many have brought her

Of hurts that wouldn't heal

Grievances unwitnessed, unaddressed

Grandmother's voice and drum

Do not extinguish these fires

But keep them burning

She dances too

And tosses handfuls of powdered herbs into the bowls of flame

Creating a light show of colored sparks

And medicinal smoke

Soon I am dancing for everyone

Who has ever brought their inflammation

To be soothed by this waterfall

Dancing a prayer

That every change they longed for

Has been cooked to fullness

In this sacred cave

Brought to life by Grandmother's breath

Imagine how Water might help you in this healing process and write out any processes with water you might engage with to nurture your ancestral healing connections. What can you add to your sacred space to remind you of the support of Water?

Mama Mermaid

By Jessica Huckabay

My dreams of breathing underwater, she tells me

Are actually ancestral memories

She has arrived in my life to remind me

Of more wisdom from the brine

It turns out that ache in my mid back

Right around my kidneys

That sometimes erupts in itchy bumps

Is a reminder of my dorsal fin

She assures me that my compulsion to live near water

Is wise

For my legs will shrivel

And my bones will become brittle

If I don't submerge myself regularly

In the sacred waters

And absorb their wisdom

She tells me of her ancestors

Who heard the call of the waters

And were given the gift of fins

And gills

As they gradually remained longer and longer

In the sea

She tells me of the constant draw to return to land

Much to their detriment

As land dwellers always seemed to want to own or destroy

What they could not understand

She reminds me of my dream

More vivid than waking reality

Of falling in love with a land dweller

And the lifetime of suffering I endured

Never able to leave the crossroads of that choice

Between my lover and the sea

She reminds me that I face similar crossroads now

And have done so many times before

At times choosing the lover

At other times choosing the sea

Always experiencing one love blossom

While the other fades

She reminds me I can hold the grief of loss

And the joy of new growth

In two hands

At the same time

I can breathe underwater

And in the air

I can sink roots into the earth

And grow fins

I can love everything and everyone

And choose a path that weaves

Closer to some and farther away from others

I can listen to my ancestors' stories

And discover that I did choose that other thread

The one I had difficulty setting down

To choose the one I followed

I chose it before

Walking in one of my ancestor's feet

Or swimming in her fins

And this is why that thread felt so familiar

So much like home

That it was hard to set it aside

I can grieve today

For that path I did not take

But when I remember my ancestors

The grief changes to celebration

For all of the stories I hold in my bones

I can celebrate the impossibility of repeating anything

Exactly

This imperative to find the new thread

Holding me to my unique path now

Imagine how Earth might support you with this ancestral healing and write out any processes or practices with Earth that you might engage with. What can you add to your sacred space to remind you of the support of Earth?

Grandmother

By Jessica Huckabay

I see you walking this land alone

Following the white dry stones pathways

Of the creek bed

Your skin brown and wrinkled

Like the cracking Earth

I hear the acorns falling

As the fall winds dance with the trees

Landing on the burnt earth you have prepared for them

I smell the smoke in your clothes

A celebration of your wisdom

Your intimacy with fire

I hear the wisdom of the elements in your voice

That does not speak words

But whispers the sounds of earth

Wind

Water

Fire

Reminding me of the true sources of wisdom

I follow you on this solitary journey

Weaving tribes together with your footsteps

Evoking visionary revelations in troubled souls

With your silence

I find you in the pause

At the bottom of my breath

In that ocean of stillness

Or dry creek bed

Or clouds passing by

Slowly changing shape while remaining the same

Drops of water suspended in air

I receive your medicine

For this ailing world

I barely recognize it

Addicted as I am

To heroic measures

But here it has been all along

This moment of allowing

This silence to emerge between breaths

This pain to motivate action

This friction to wear down the sharp edges that divide us

This instinct for survival to arise from deep within us

This collapse to our knees

To unlock the flow of miraculous regeneration

I feel the patience in your presence

A grandmother's patience

A grandmother who knows

What other's experience as the end

Of her life

Of a way of life

Is only the beginning

What others experience as a loss of power

Of agency

Death

Is a portal to great power

And when others long for speed

I feel you resting

Following the pace of nature

The most potent change maker alive

I feel the storms of change

Brewing in your belly

I feel the power of your rage

Ravaging this unsustainability

Like wildfire

Clearing the way for the acorns

To drop onto scorched soil once more

To nourish us through the winter

I feel your smile

And take your hand

As you reach for me through the smoke

Leading me to hidden places

Revealing new wisdoms

I am only now ready to receive

How does this poem inspire you?

Imagine how Air can support you on your healing journey and write out any processes and/or practices with Air that might nurture you that you feel inspired to explore. What objects can you bring into your sacred space to remind you of the support of Air?

I felt as if I could feel the blood, womb, and life force of different energies like never before- a higher, darker cosmic energy.

Not negative, just black like the emptiness of space, but it's not empty at all. It's fertile, ready, and constantly making love with energies- then all that is in the cosmos give birth to planets, life, rock, movement, light, and welcomes the energy of death as stars shrink and expand to die like each breath we take.

The energy of death is released back into the darkness to fuel new life- un, sub, and conscious. It's like a casing, like the womb, only this is not the only one. There are multiple wombs.

Like women standing side by side, and all around each other infinitely. Then, there is Earthly. The broad. The Lady in waiting has been fertilized and now being tossed aside and destroyed.

In Old times, the Elders were respected, now, with Capitalism, corporations and western influences, the elders in our culture are not respected. They are dismissed, tossed away, and their wisdom destroyed.

I see Earth in her Crone age. A wearing out abused mother who is aged and tired. She's a massive force, but when she sees what's happening, does she even want to fight back? If she gives up, we're fucked. She knows that. It's like right now, she's with that.

But, it's our blood. Women's blood returning to the Earth that will help her heal, remember, and make the decision. Jennifer

Imagine how Fire might support your healing journey and write out any processes/practices with Fire that might nurture you. What objects might you bring into your sacred space to remind you of the support of Fire?

What is your relationship with Divine energy like? Are there any Divine Beings that you feel connected with? What is your relationship with them like? How do you embody their essence?

What human cultures do the Divine Beings you connect with come from? How does your ancestral heritage relate to the cultures these Divine Beings come from? Is there any healing to be engaged with between your ancestral heritage and the cultural heritage of these Divine Beings?

If you feel connected mostly with Divine Beings from outside of your ancestral cultural heritage, what research might you do to find out more about your Divine cultural heritage? Write out a conversation with your ancient wisdom ancestor asking them to guide you to reconnect with your Divine cultural heritage.

Divine Mother's Recipe for Me

By Jessica Huckabay

Getting the recipe for my life from Divine Mother

Has been no easy task

I sit in rapt devotion to her movements

On a wicker bar stool at the edge of her tiled kitchen counter

Listening to her stories and asking questions

Each time she goes rummaging in her cupboards

For another obscure ingredient to add to the great bowl

That is my life

I must hold a measuring cup out

Underneath the stream of what she is pouring in

Capturing it as it falls

To discover how much she is adding

I have already written down

A drugged cockful of irresponsibility

Plus a 17-year-old woman full of reproductive ignorance

Mix together with vigor

For as long as it takes for conception to occur

Remove all further ingredients the man might contribute

And let sit in the warm dark oven of family secrecy

Don't let anyone know it is rising

Their awareness might ruin it

Once risen, add a gallon of profit oriented medical intervention

Punch down that round belly

With a syringe full of epidural

Kneed that baby out

And separate her from her mother for 4 hours

Withhold the rich colostrum

And the halo of the golden hour

No matter how much she and the mother cry for each other

Let this longing fill both with and infinite dose of fierce love

And a pinch of siren song

Not too much though

For vocal suppression is an essential ingredient

To later develop into the full flavors of liberation

Add much less breast milk than is natural

Once you bring them back together

Replacing it with allergen filled experimental formula

Make sure to include the misinformation about breastfeeding

To disrupt the mother's natural instincts

When the child becomes sick with diarrhea for a month

Almost dying in her first year of life

Add cool aid to keep her hydrated

And further thwart her digestive health

Cultivating her addiction to processed sugar

Be sure to remedy this briefly with several years full of devotion

To PB n J's made whole grain breads and unsweetened peanut butter and fruit spreads

She will most likely trade these for twinkies at school

But they will plant seeds of desire

For the healthy diet she will require later in life

And be sure to add a 15-year dose of adoption papers

And mix in the regular yelling matches

Developing the fibers of her prayers

Place in a preheated society on the brink of self-annihilation

Checking every 27 years

Against this complex geometry of stars and planets

Arranged just so

Poking here and here

Where Saturn activates her purpose

And bless her regularly with Goddess journals and dreams

Falling off the shelves in used book stores

And in the night

Edging her away from the shape of the mold you poured her into

Breathe your joy and unconditional love regularly onto her golden-brown skin

As her face turns towards your brilliance

Ever more permanently

After 47 years or so she will stop looking anywhere else

That's when you know she is done

Serve hot and enjoy

Imagine that you can connect with a Divine Being who is intimately connected with your ancestral cultural heritage right now. Imagine your womb wisdom can show you what they look like, what they feel like, what wisdom and healing they have to offer you. Write about them. Write out a conversation with them asking them any questions you feel to ask to get to know them.

Imagine that a council came together to meet with your soul before you were conceived to celebrate your choice to incarnate into this lifetime. Included in this council were your ancient wisdom ancestor(s), divine beings intimate with the cultural heritage lineages you would enter into, wisdom allies, and any ancestors who had gifts, wisdom, and requests for you as you entered into this lifetime. Imagine that each member of this council brought you a gift that became part of your soul purpose in this life. Describe meeting the members of this council as you imagine it might have been and any ceremonial activities that may have occurred. Write about the gifts each council member brought you and what aspects of your soul purpose each gift represented.

How have your experiences in your life supported the soul purpose wisdom your pre-conception council initiated with you?

Conception

What was your parents' relationship like when you were conceived? If you don't know, imagine what it might have been like based on what you do know about them. Write a story about how you imagine the time they spent together might have been like leading up to and following your conception. Go into as much detail as you can.

Were your parents planning on getting pregnant together when your conception occurred? Imagine what their intentions were around conception when they were preparing to be intimate together. Write a story imagining and describing what both of them were thinking and feeling leading up to your conception and afterwards.

What were the circumstances of your actual conception? Was it a happy, pleasure filled union? Or something else? Imagine what those intimate moments were like for both of your parents and write a story about it. Embellish this story with sensory details. What were the tastes, smells, textures, temperatures, sounds, images, and emotions of the encounter.

Was your birth parent orgasmic during the sexual encounter that resulted in your conception? If you do not know, what do you imagine to be true? Write a story about how you imagine your birth parent's sexual arousal and emotions to have been during this encounter. Write another story about your other parent's experiences of sexual arousal during your conception.

The Myth of Immaculate Conception

By Jessica Huckabay

My mother struggled

Searching for the joys

Of human womanhood

Amidst myths of original sin

These myths claimed that just being conceived

Was an act of evil

And being born

Through the female birth canal

Made us all unworthy

Of divine love

Especially women

For being in possession of

A birth canal

A womb

We needed to prove our worthiness

Endlessly

By prostration in service

And subjection to abuse

And any enjoyment

Of our female anatomy

Was proof

Of our unworthiness and separation

From God

My mother's initiation into womanhood

Fertility, sexuality

Came from my grandmother

Showing her to use her sexuality

To gain power

In the world of male domination

She found herself lost in the void

Between vixen and virgin

That is where she plucked me

From the tree of ignorance, shame, and grief

Growing in a dark corner of the mystery

Whose agony evoked

The compassion of my soul

She was drawn to my soul

Like a moth to light

Longing for the gifts I brought

Familiar with my flavors and aromas

We had shared womb space before

She knew the importance of her role

Without knowing

She protected me from abortion

Kept me a secret

Held to the only thread of truth

She could find amidst the myths and lies

That structured her life

"Life is sacred"

This knowing pulsed

A message from Divine Mother

Beaming clear through the fog

Of trauma induced cacophony

"Life is sacred

Motherhood is a precious gift

Protect this treasure

At all costs"

Her heart and womb

Unified

With the drumbeat

Of this imperative

Guiding her through the dark nights

Of solitude

Fear

Sorrow

That were to come

With no solace offered

From the Beaver Cleaver

White Washed reality

Surrounding her lonely ache

Her living mantra

Silently gestating

Her one source of hope

One precious gift

One gleaming miracle

Me

Awakening the strongest

Unconditional love

That will ever exist

Motherly love

Guiding her through the darkness

Of deception

Betrayal

Abuse

Solitude

To the power of love

Again and again

Unbeknownst to her

She became that beacon

Of infinite love

Arising out of nowhere

Lighting up that darkness

Bringing the balm of pleasure

To the deepest hurts

Lighting the spark of laughter

In the driest tallest piles of lies

Setting fire to the ruins

Of these perfect lives

We were supposed to be living

Lighting up the night

With the joy

Rising from the ashes of our pain

Revealing the truth of her worth

Secretly gestating in the darkness

All these years

The truth of all conception finally revealed

As immaculate

For each life is precious

Each journey perfect

In its imperfection

Each birth blessed

With Infinite Motherly Love

When did your parents discover that the conception had occurred? How did they feel about it? If you don't know, imagine how this discovery might have taken place and how they felt about it and write it out.

In what ways did your conception create a blueprint for your life? What recurring patterns of behavior, experience, energy, health, or emotion do you notice might originate from this conception experience?

How would you like to revise this conception experience and the blueprint it provided for your life? What energies would you like to include more of in this revised conception you are imagining? What energies would you like to include less of?

Imagine that you could travel back in time and revisit the moments leading up to and following your conception and somehow infuse the cells that developed into you with the energies you want to add and shield them from the energies you want less of. Which of your pre-conception council allies might help you with this process? Describe a ceremony or process you might offer your cellular self with the help of these allies.

Immaculate Re-conception

A message from Mother Mary

By Jessica Huckabay

About that statue of me you have on your altar

The one you got from the thrift store

To reclaim and rescue my memory...

Thank you for your love

For hearing my call of despair

Languishing under the weight of the lies about me

And for listening to my voice

Firstly, the color of my skin

On the statue

Is all wrong

My skin was and is much darker

So dark my eyes gleamed like stars

In the night

The flowing robes with gold edges are good

But the sunburst halo behind my head

Is a bit imbalanced, don't you think?

There needs to be at least two more

And the biggest one in front of my womb

The one behind my heart is a bit too small

And the burning flames rising could be bigger as well

One at my power center to represent my integrity

Fortitude, and stamina

And the one at my womb

That womb you worship with prayers

Grateful for its fruits

How about a cornucopia

Overflowing with nourishment

There as well?

As for the story so many are telling

About my virginity

That word meant something different to us back then

It just meant that I wasn't beholden to any man

I was free to love as I chose

And I chose to love

I made love to the divine

In all my lovers

They were all angels

But one in particular

Gleamed in the night

I sang songs about our union

We blossomed in divine love together

Our lovemaking ignited a love so great in me

You are still blessed by it

Many millennia hence

It was so brilliant

So alive

That my son was conceived

His conception was an explosion of divine bliss

He was the son of the embodiment of divine love

That was our union

So yes, he was the Son of God

But not because I did not have sex with a human man

But because our sex was divine

It grieves my heart

To see the suffering humans have created

By perpetuating this misconception

By equating sexuality with sin

By making God asexual

This is so obviously a lie

All life is created sexually

If God created all life

How could God be asexual?

So I thank you for reclaiming

Your sexuality as one of Gods most precious gifts

And for recognizing that it is the union of God and Goddess

Within each of us

And between us

That creates new life

Yes I suffered and forgave much

And can teach you pure divine unconditional motherly love

Nurturing you from the passion of my heart

Through the milk of my breasts

And from the fruits of my womb

Which are not limited to my beautiful son

Who lived in divine union

Because that was how he was conceived

But pour forth as the fruits of emotional wisdom

Teaching you how your sexuality

Can nourish your creativity

How your monthly cycles can help you

Shed lies and illness

And activate magical rhythms and codes of artistry

How your embodied and rooted divine love

From the womb

Can create miraculous healing

For all of humanity

Nourishing our evolution

Towards our purpose as a species

Embodying heaven here on earth

So yes, light a candle, or a thousand

For your prayers to me

And then go and awaken your womb

Reclaim your sex

Embody the divine light of your essence

Re-conceive of yourself

As a divine being fully integrating into your human form

Transforming humanity with every breath

With every orgasm

With every creative passion that arises in you

That you nourish and bring to fruition

Imagining that the Fruits of my Womb

Pouring forth

Nourish your womb to pour forth as well

Not just brilliant children

But divine love

Genius

Miracles

Healing

Transformation

Evolution

Heaven here on Earth

Gestation

Describe any information you have about the first few weeks of your gestation time in your birth parent's womb, from stories you have been told by your parents and family, and/or from what you remember/imagine. Write a story about what you imagine experiencing as you developed during that first week.

Describe any emotional and/or energetic feelings you have about these early weeks of your gestation. Are there any surprising feelings you are encountering while reflecting on this time?

Describe any insights, gifts, inspirations, or guidance the element of Air might have for you around this gestation time and for your life.

How might you integrate the wisdom of the element Air into your daily life? Are there any practices that particularly inspire you to engage with more frequently? Please describe.

I keep thinking about breath. The first breath at birth, how we transfer our life dependency from the umbilical connection to the rhythm of breathing, which is a huge paradigm shift, from continuous supply to learning to take in and then trust to breathe out, let go, become empty. It's a very profound change.

I have been researching ancient names of the goddess in different languages. There seems to be a root name that begins with a vowel, has a sound in the middle that is difficult to spell or pronounce and seems to be a kind of back of the throat sound, and another vowel at the end. I've been trying to figure out the essence of this name, and then at a shamanic circle people were saying "aho". I realized that this word, and the name of the goddess are the sound of breath, breathe in, ah, breathe out, ha. The goddess of Life has this name, ...Isis /Wadjet , Akka, Hecate, and many more are variations that have been distorted through time and translation.
Pennifer Moonmama

The freedom I felt reminded me of the purity of my soul. Nothing can stain it. I am always free no matter what conditioning I have acquired or what traumas I have endured. Anata

Imagine inviting your pre-conception council allies to support you in offering beneficial influences to your gestating self during the first week of your development. What energies, gifts, or emotions might you want to bath yourself in at that time? How might you like to support your parents?

Please describe any information you have about the later part of your first trimester and the first part of your second trimester of your gestation time in your birth parent's womb, from stories you have been told by your parents and family, and/or from what you remember/imagine.

Please describe any emotional and/or energetic feelings you have about this time of your gestation. Are there any surprising feelings you are encountering while reflecting on this time?

Please describe any insights, gifts, inspirations, or guidance the element of Water might have for you around this gestation time and for your life.

Flow, ease, bubbles! Donna-Lee Ida

How might you integrate the wisdom of the element of Water into your daily life? Are there any practices that particularly inspire you to engage with more frequently? Please describe.

All waters--the sea, waterfalls, rivers, streams, rain, hot springs, pools--all converged and transformed before my eyes into droplets of blessings full of life and love. Indira

Imagine you invite your pre-conception council allies to support you in nourishing your gestating self and your parents during this time of your gestation. How do you imagine bringing beneficial energies and influences into your development at this time with the help of your allies? Describe a ceremony or process you imagine doing together.

The blessings of the womb waters from the Dolphins also called in Angels who transmuted the "toxic" waters into clear, beautiful, shining nourishment. Indira

Please describe any information you have about the later part of your second trimester and the first part of your third trimester of your gestation time in your birth parent's womb, from stories you have been told by your parents and family, and/or from what you remember/imagine.

Please describe any emotional and/or energetic feelings you have about this time of your gestation. Are there any surprising feelings you are encountering while reflecting on this time?

Please describe any insights, gifts, inspirations, or guidance the element of Fire might have for you around this gestation time and for your life.

Fire burns through the bullshit. It is focus, direction, action. Fire sees and moves toward, unapologetically. I am knowing and claiming my strength from the focus of fire and burning off excess thoughts and energy. Thalia

How might you integrate the wisdom of the element Fire into your daily life? Are there any practices that particularly inspire you to engage with more frequently? Please describe.

Imagine visiting this gestational time with your pre-conception council allies and nurturing your developing self as well as your parents. What beneficial energies, feelings, and influences might you bring to offer to yourself? Describe a ceremony or process you might do together to infuse this time with more beneficial energies and influences.

Please describe any information you have about the last part of your gestation time in your birth parent's womb, from stories you have been told by your parents and family, and/or from what you remember/imagine.

Please describe any emotional and/or energetic feelings you have about this time of your gestation. Are there any surprising feelings you are encountering while reflecting on this time?

Please describe any insights, gifts, inspirations, or guidance the element of Earth might have for you around this gestation time and for your life.

I feel that is why I chose to be born as an Aires sign, the first one in horoscope order. That's where I also have my drive to go against the wall with my head if it needs be. I love my highly vivid energy and fiery nature, but also felt trapped and restrained by the womb as a baby for instance. I found it difficult to relax in the dark nourishing womb, until I found my entrance to the WYRD field two years ago. Wyrd to me is this void, the dark womb of the mother. When I chant HUUUUL, which stands for cave and resembles the vibration of the dark womb, I can relax into the void and embrace the miracles from the dark. Erika

How might you integrate the wisdom of the element Earth into your daily life? Are there any practices that particularly inspire you to engage with more frequently? Please describe.

I am celebrating the real physicality of my body, as if it feels more real than it used to. My body connected to the earth, magnetically attached, the earth feels secure, she's not going to let me go. I can resonate with the deep slow rhythm if the earth, she lets me take my time.
Pennifer Moonmama

Imagine inviting your pre-conception council allies to support you in bringing beneficial energies, feelings, and influences to you and your parents during the last part of your gestation. What gifts might you bring? Describe a blessing ceremony you might offer yourself and your family in preparation for your birth.

Please write out an account of your birth parent's pregnancy with you. How were they feeling about being pregnant? What kind of support did they have? If you don't know, write out what you imagine to be true based on what you do know.

Was there another parent involved in your development during gestation in any way? Did they talk with you? Were they providing for your birth parent? Supporting them? How were they anticipating your birth?

What was the overall emotional quality of your gestational period? Did your birth parent feel happy to be pregnant? Did they feel stressed?

Were there any stressful events that occurred for your birth parent during your gestation? Please describe.

How do you feel the emotional quality of your gestation influenced your development? Your life?

Birth

Please write out an account of how you were born.

How was your birth parent feeling throughout the birth process? Emotionally? Physically? Spiritually? If you don't have a first-hand account from them, how do you imagine they would answer this question?

Was there another parent present at your birth? How did they participate? How were they feeling during the birth? If you don't have a first-hand account from them, how do you imagine they would answer these questions?

Who else was present at your birth besides your parent(s) and yourself? What energy signature do you feel they contributed to your life?

Were there any medical interventions in your birth process? How did these affect your birth experience?

Did you have immediate skin to skin contact and bonding with your parents when you were born? How do you feel this affect your development one way or the other?

Did your start breastfeeding right away after being born? How do you feel this affected you one way or the other?

What feelings come up for you as you reflect on these questions? How do you feel to nurture yourself and tend to these feelings right now?

I've always had abandonment issues and issues surrounding trust. I had a memory come up before going to sleep last night about a dog we had when I was 3. She was a beautiful female Collie and she was so loving towards my sister and I, she would lay down and let us use her as a pillow and tie bonnets on her head. However, she ran away and I was heartbroken. I didn't realize how that had affected me until last night when the memory came back. She was a very nurturing, mothering presence in my early life, even though she was a dog, she embodied Divine Mothers love. I think she came last night to tell me how sorry she was for abandoning us like that. She herself was heartbroken and missed her family, the one who had given her up, so much that she kept running away to try and get back to them, she was so worried about them. She did not mean to hurt us, she was just so full of grief she didn't know what else to do. She wanted me to know she loved us but the bonds with her other family were very strong. Lila

Are there any important aspects of birth that you feel were missing for you? If so, how might you imagine bringing those missing aspects if you could travel back in time and fill in those gaps? Imagine inviting your pre-conception council allies to support you in a re-birthing ceremony in which you created a birth process for yourself that gave you everything you needed to fulfill your soul purpose. Describe that ceremony.

Letter to my Mother's Womb

By Jessica Huckabay

Dear lost sanctuary of my mother's womb

Thank you for nurturing me

Filling me with life

Keeping me hidden from those who would have terminated my existence

While giving me the space and freedom to learn how to move on my own

Thank you for radiating my love, wisdom, and assurance to my mother's heart and mind

 As she navigated the impossible obstacles to this pregnancy

Thank you for delivering all of her feelings to me

So I could know exactly what medicine to become

And thank you for giving me just the right firmness to kick my legs against

When it was time for me to emerge

Mistressfully untangling what belongs to me from what belongs to her

While opening so gracefully

Giving my mother so much pleasure during my passage out of her

And thank you for continuing to radiate nourishment

Broadcasting motherly love out into the hospital corridors

So I could hear her voice calling for me

Feel her passion to care for me

Feel her touch in the touch of the nurses as they washed me

Feel her rage protecting me, drawing me back to her

Thank you for igniting that fire within her, that fire within me

I can still feel your silken red walls surrounding me

The cord feeding me through my navel, though it has been long ago discarded

And though I had to wait too long for those first sips of her sweet milk

And only got a short taste before this world dried her up

And gave me sickening substitutes

Thank you for stepping in with your rich flow of wisdom

Meeting each disappointment

Each fearful encounter

Each aching challenge

Each desperate longing

With a knowing that all is well

That there is a deeper purpose to this suffering

And that I am infinitely loved despite the constant onslaught of this love stopping world

Thank you for delivering ancient wisdom

From before these self-destructive

Womb silencing human habits started to develop

And awakening me to your power that I carry within me

Thank you for teaching me how to develop these powers in myself

Thank you for opening my voice to transmit this awakening to the world.

Re-Parenting

Please share about what you know about your experience as an infant. Were you breastfed? For how long? How do you feel this influenced your development? What blueprint did it create for you in your life?

Were your parents supported to be with you and focus all of her attention on bonding with you for the first months after you were born? If not, what did they have to do instead? How do you feel this influenced your development? What blueprint did this create for you in your life?

Were your parents under any stress during your infancy and childhood? Either low grade chronic stress or any bigger acute stressful situations? If so, how do you feel this influenced your development? What blueprints did this create for your life?

My Mother's Love

By Jessica Huckabay

The smell of my mother's love

Conjured out of the smoke and mirrors

The lies that told her she had nothing of value

Out of her own bone marrow

She produced this richness

From the bottom of the pit of poverty

It hurt her deeply

Stripping her of vital nutrients

For she put her own essence into it

With no way to replenish it readily at hand

I could feel her unmet need behind this gift of life she gave me

I could taste the gaps between what she knew to give and my own needs

I found a way to give back to her, to fill those gaps

In hopes we could both be freed from this trap

This looping of emptiness feeding upon itself

I didn't realize at first

That this emptiness was the source

That at that darkest point of disappointment

The greatest invisible power resides

Great Mother's footsteps find purchase

In that emptiness

In those gaps

Where her children's needs fall through

That is where her hands always are

Fingers plump and held securely together

Cupped

To catch what we think we lost

What we imagined we missed

She steps into our own bodies

Offering her breasts

Pressed into the underside of our nipples

As we attempt to breastfeed our inner infant

Retroactively

Resentful that our mother couldn't

Didn't know

Was misinformed

Her voluptuous sweet milk

Flows through our hearts

Bathing the anger

In her eternal presence

We realize that there she was

All along

Stepping into the gaps in our mothers' bodies

Our grandmothers' bodies

She is the only reason we are still miraculously alive

Given all of the lies about how life works flying around

She strings a web, silvery grey sinews

Elastic strength

Through our chest

And like a great spider, she feels the twanging

Twitching struggle

When our anger, our fear, our sadness gets caught there

Pulling our shoulder blades against our ribs

Squeezing and crowding our hearts and lungs

This is when she jumps down

With pointed toes at the bottom of her infinite plumpness

And bounces with jubilation

Sending all of these heart guests

Into the air

In arcs of laughter and lightness

Anger still manages to maintain a scowl

But she knows she can rage whenever she likes

In Great Mothers unconditional embrace

Sadness' tears forget what they were about

And grief takes the opportunity

To bounce through her multiple identities

Switching places with all the others repeatedly

All comes to rest in laughter

And storytelling

Sometimes Great Mother listens

Weaving the threads of our sensory journeys

Into the fabric of life she tends so lovingly

Other times she speaks, sings, dances Her stories

Enrapturing us with possibility

Pleasure, healing, wisdom, love

Planting the seeds of her presence

In the darkness of our wombs

Where we can forget and remember

Again and again

Until the way is no longer bumpy

But bouncy and blissful

And we find ourselves sitting on her lap

Wordless

Barely taking up the space on one of her thighs

Surrounded and infused by her blue green peace

Smelling it in our clothes the rest of the day.

What would you say the strongest emotions your parents felt while parenting you were? How do you feel these emotions influenced your development? What blueprints did they create for your life?

What was your parents' relationship like during your infancy and early childhood? How do you feel this influenced your development? What blueprints did this create for your life?

What were your parents' relationships with their parents like? How do you feel this influenced your development? What blueprints did this create for your life?

What emotional wisdom do you feel you absorbed from your parents during your infancy and childhood? Did they model any healthy, wise ways of relating and living in the world? If so, how did this influence your development? What blueprints did this create for your life?

A Conversation with my Divine/Human Mother

By Jessica Huckabay

My mother lived her life on top of an emptiness. She found love and devoted herself to it as medicine for this emptiness. She found ways to give love despite the cruelty and taking she experienced from all around her. A thread of magic, a fruit bearing vine wove through her whole being, including the emptiness. The vine grows thorny and dry as it passes through the emptiness, but its roots managed to find cracks in the concrete structures boxing her out of vibrance where just enough moisture, just enough nourishment managed to gather. She learned how to breathe nourishment out of thin air. She learned that simple water is the most important thing to drink and managed to keep life flowing through her vine of love with a constant drip of simple water, no added sweeteners or colors, just the pure clear water, mostly just from the tap. No treks to the spring or fancy bottled water, and sometimes just breathing it out of thin air.

Mom, I want to say that it is time to find the spring that flows abundantly, filling that emptiness. It is time to overflow instead of rasp and eek. It is time to swim in the ocean instead of wiping condensation off of the windows to rub on your skin. It is time to receive the fruits of all you have poured into this vine of love, feeding others with what it produces. It is time to curl up at the roots of this vine and let the flower petals and leaves caresse you, love you. It is time to ask for what you need, for what you want, and give yourself permission to receive. It is time to recognize the lies that said you could give more to your loved ones if you neglected yourself. It is time to discover how to be in balance with this love.

Mom, I want to say that the bottom of your well has always been there, that the water was not the danger. The danger was in the giving too much so the water level was constantly dropping. And now you lie in a heap at the bottom of that well, dry stones surrounding you.

Mom, I want to say I can help you crack open the stone that is covering your spring. It's right there, the one in the middle of the bottom of you. It just needs a little nudge to come loose. You can use it to close up the overly large holes that have drained your well before it ever had the chance to fill up. I invite you to rest and float on the water as it rises. Let the water fill you. Let it raise you up into the sunlight. Let it bath you, give you visions of silvery moonlight and tree branches dancing with the stars. Let it carry you down the river where we can sit together and laugh.

Mom, it is time to celebrate this flow of life that brought you to the bottom so you would remember how to love yourself. It is time to listen to the whisper of wisdom that is that spring flowing in, refilling you, guiding you, showing you your purpose.

Helping you bring the darkness of the bottom of the well, potent medicine, to those who need it. May we hear it in the echo of your voice that still remains, even when you return to fullness. May we hear your story, your song, and feel the importance of this medicine. Reminding us of the lies that we must scrape and scrub off of our skin, scour from our bones, flush out from our brains and bellies. Reminding us that the emptiness at the bottom of the well is a place to visit and remember, but not to dwell in. It is a place to hold and carry the flow of the fullness of life.

For as we live, we can engage with this fullness, this overflowing of life. If we seek emptiness too much, like those who reject the 10,000 things in favor of liberation, or give too much without replenishing, we soon find ourselves facing the ultimate passage out of life, into another world. Death awaits us at the threshold of emptiness. We will all meet death there eventually. For now, Mom, I want to say, let's live.

Mom, I want you to tell me, show me, guide me along the way. Your infinite wisdom flashes within me at the bottom of my breath and all around me in the uncurling petals of roses and poppies, in the fattening lupine seeds, offering food for every hungry corner of me. Tell me where that magic elixir is, the one I can feed to the whole world at once and stop the suffering. Show me how to save us from our own folly. Teach me how to find freedom from my own delusions and stay in that freedom for good.

Please tell me that my efforts to follow what I think you are telling me are on track, that I have heard your guidance clearly and am implementing it well. Please tell me the fruits of my labors will ripen quickly and have the beneficial nourishing effect I want them to have for me and everyone.

No, don't tell me that. I don't want to hear that. Yes, I know you have told me this before, that the mystery has no guarantees, and that the world is wild, life is wild, that your will cannot be tamed, that my capacities to understand are limited, that if you instantly removed all of my delusions and delivered me into permanent freedom, the shock would destroy me. I do not want to hear that I will have to learn by living which includes fumbling around with mistakes, misdirection, and tricks, turning lies over and over on my tongue to get so familiar with the flavor before I remember that I can spit. I know I already know this, you have told me all of this before. I don't want to hear this again. This is why I am asking you to tell me the other things.

And no, I don't want you to lie to me. Yes, I know that the wisdom of resting, digesting, gestating in the darkness of the unknown has always delivered unexpected fruits. I just want to know for sure that it will again, this time, now. And don't laugh at me. I know I am an adult woman throwing a temper tantrum about the truth I already know. I just want you to take away the pain, the suffering, now. It seems we have had enough. It seems you are saying you have had enough. So please tell me how we can stop this self-perpetuating pain.

Please.

Mom?

Don't go giving me the silent treatment. Just because you have already told me the exact wisdom I am begging you for and now I just have to spend my precious life grappling with how to live it, just because I agreed to this endeavor generations ago and read the fine print about how the gifts of a life at this time in human evolution would come with some significant costs. And yes, I read the no returns policy on human incarnation as well. Please stop gazing at me so softly, with such loving eyes, silently grinning at my anguish. Give me the way out! The solution! Fix this!

Aaahhhgggghhh!

Yes, I know. It is here inside me. This being. This feeling. This discomfort, dissatisfaction, desperation, anguish. I know that if you took those things away it would prevent me from finding that which I seek. I know. I know. And yes, I am complaining when you tell me the very thing I begged you to tell me. I just don't like that answer. There must be another way. Where is the way of pleasure? The way of joy? The way of truth and abundant flowing milk and honey? Now I am longing for just the right things you say? Like my longing is supposed to make it happen? Exactly? What is that supposed to mean? Exactly that? That my longing will make it happen? Just as simple as that?

So you are saying my desire is the very answer I am longing for, the longing itself is the medicine for itself. That can't be true. If that were true, then I would be my own medicine too. That everything that hurt would contain the medicine it needs within itself. That every problem contains its own solution.

Exactly? There you go again, making me answer my own questions. How can you abandon me like that? Leave me to my own devices?

What? What do you mean who's voice do I think I am hearing from within me telling me these answers. That was all my voice. Or was it you speaking through me? How did you get in here? How did you...Mom!!!

What unhealthy emotional patterns do you feel you learned from your parents during your infancy and childhood? How did their lack of emotional wisdom influence your development? What blueprints did this create in your life?

Do you implement any of your parents' emotional wisdom and strengths in your life? Please describe. Is there any of their wisdom you would like to implement more?

Do you repeat any of your parents' unwise, unhealthy emotional patterns in your life? Please describe. How would you like to be less like them?

If you could have had the ideal parent(s) with all of the qualities you are grateful they had, plus all of the qualities you wish they had, what would they be like? Please describe in detail, including all of the emotional wisdom patterns you did receive from them and the ones you wished you had.

If your parents had had a direct line to Divine Parents, and had been fully supported by them to implement Divine Womb Wisdom in their parenting, what would have been different for you during your infancy and childhood?

If a Divine Parent was guiding you right now to become the parent you never had, bringing their wisdom to yourself at all of the points in your childhood that you feel you needed more quality parenting, what would they guide you to do? What ages would you revisit with their guidance in place? How would you re-parent yourself?

Imagine that you travel to a sacred Womb Garden where your inner child resides. What does this garden look like? What plants are growing there? What condition are they in? Do they need any care from you?

Imagine that you meet your inner child in this womb garden. Where do you meet them? What part of the garden are they in? How do they appear? What are they wearing? What age are they? How do they feel?

Imagine that the Water element has some gifts for you and your inner child in this Womb garden. Describe these watery gifts and any process or journey Water takes you and your inner child on. Describe any changes you feel in yourself and your inner child from this interaction with Water.

Goddess Isis appeared she spoke to me about the gift of vulnerability and how tears are of the same composition as our womb water when we are babies the ones we swim in, how vulnerability is softness and softness is strength if I changed my perception of it. Isis

Imagine that you meet a Divine Parent in your Womb Garden and they are holding and nurturing your inner infant, meeting any unmet needs your inner infant experienced during your infancy. Describe how this Divine Parent is caring for your inner infant.

Imagine that there are beneficial herbal plant allies in your Womb Garden. What qualities do they have? Are they herbs that you are familiar with? How do they support you and your inner child?

Pink Hibiscus was the flower nurturing me the most. The wisdom was to always come back to this flower as the staple of the island's love for supporting and strengthen life. Ferns. There were different types and various sizes of ferns all around. The ferns were my shelter and part of my bed. It's where I had comfort. The ferns told me all things are possible. That the curls were the spiral, the symbols of the Goddess reminding me of the Goddess within myself. The Goddess and I commune and are part of each other. The opened ferns were the Goddesses opening her magic of her prayers blessing the Earth and all of those who are supported from it. The ferns kept me soft, protected, regulated and comforted. Jennifer

Imagine that there are beneficial animals in your Womb Garden. Which animals are there for you? How do they support you and your inner child?

There were white birds. The wisdom: Songs are flight upward and into freedom. Soar in hymns and music. The songs of the mother come in many voices. There are different sounds for everything, but the notes are what makes the difference. Jennifer

Imagine there are other beneficial allies in your Womb Garden, perhaps ancestors, divine beings, angels, mystical beings, knowing that you are surrounded by your Wise Womb Membrane that only allows beneficial energies into your sanctuary. Describe the allies that might be there to support you and your inner child and how they do so.

The path was of that of "kalaripayattu", a martial art I am learning. It had an oil lamp, deity and weapons. It led to a forest with a river nearby. The gate was made of glass when I looked closely it was made of bones, it was sturdy. The priestess Deity with me was the fanged Goddess green Tara and the guardian of the gate was Palden Lhamo (Tibetan equivalent of Goddess Kali). I was required to be a mother to enter or have mothering energy. I saw a birth pool there and a guy I have a crush on who was waiting to help me birth. I saw copper pots filled with water. At one point I saw a baby clinging to my body. She radiated out of my body and my body started to glow. My breasts became fuller and radiant and milk started to glow. I grew fangs too. I felt powerful. My inner child drank heartily and my mother felt forgiven. Dr. Sneha Rooh

Imagine there are flowers blooming in your Womb Garden. Do you recognize these flowers? Describe them in detail and write about how they might support you and your inner child.

Imagine that the herbs and flowers in your Womb Garden can speak to you and teach you how you can make medicine with them. Write out your conversation with them.

Write about any memories you have from your childhood when you experienced a sense of strong awareness about your parents or yourself that your parents did not seem to share.

Were you passionate about anything uniquely yours during your childhood? Please describe what that was and how you felt about it.

Art. It was the only thing that I could do that couldn't be controlled by anyone else. It was all my own and gave me my own space and allowed me the freedom to express my creativity in any way I chose. I liked that it was one place in my life where there didn't seem to be any rules and I could live outside the box, where I was genuinely most comfortable. Lila

Did your parents, other family members, and teachers/mentors support you around your passions? Did they ever undermine, criticize, judge, or discourage you from exploring your passions, desires, and dreams? Please describe your memories of this support and/or discouragement you received.

What kind of role modeling was available to you about pursuing your passions and creative dreams? Were your parents fulfilled in their creativity or did they sacrifice it for financial security? How did you feel about this growing up? How do you feel about this now?

Do you have any childhood passions that you had to abandon or smother in order to meet life's demands? Are any of them still smoldering and longing to be rekindled? Please describe what you loved about these childhood passions and how you might rekindle them now.

Is there any way you wish your parents, teachers, and mentors might have supported you more towards fulfilling your childhood dreams? Is there anything you wish they had said or done for you to give you permission to fully develop into your purpose? How can you give this support to yourself now?

Imagine that you revisit your Womb Garden where your inner child resides. How have things changed there since your last visit?

Imagine the element of Fire has some gifts for you and your inner child in your Womb Garden. Describe these gifts and any journey you go on guided by the element of Fire.

Imagine that there are beneficial allies in your Womb Garden that support your passionate self-expression and fulfillment of your desires. How do these allies interact with you and your inner child? What gifts do they bring you? What journeys do they take you on?

Imagine there are herbal and flower allies in your Womb Garden that have particular medicine for you to support your passionate self-expression and fulfillment of your desires. What plants might these be? Write out conversations with these plants in which they instruct you on how to make herbal preparations to support yourself in this way.

Please share about any of your experiences as a young child that you feel were deeply influential in your emotional development. What strengths did those experiences help you develop? How did those experiences limit your development?

Imagine that you visit the Womb Garden again and the element of Air has gifts and wisdom for you and your inner child. Write about these gifts from Air and how you and your inner child experience them. How do these gifts benefit you?

During the meditation my two power spirit birds raven and hummingbird were with me, flying through the air element with great messages to me. The raven is my great ally which I am also currently painting... The raven used to be white but has become black through so many dark messages and imprints from us humans which she carries back and forth between worlds. She had the message for me that when I dive deep and incorporate all my shadows, I am similarly whole and the paradox between white and black dissolves.

The Hummingbird similarly dissolves paradoxes and brings me joy and love. I found out that the Hummingbird is my mentor archetype embodying the essence of love, joy and unity. Those energies were very present with me during the meditation and I could feel unconditional love throughout my whole body. I can see immediate connections between the meditation and my everyday life, because ALL my senses are sharpened and I have the feeling of seeing and perceiving the world with multiple eyes and senses. I can see signs and symbols all over and can directly communicate with my spirit guides. Erika

Imagine that the element of Air has some instructions for you about how to process any unresolved emotions you might still be carrying from your childhood. What does Air have to teach you about this? What practices does Air show you and your inner child that you can do together to heal from any difficult experiences you may have had growing up?

Imagine that beneficial allies also arrive in your Womb Garden to help you and your inner child with any healing processes you need to engage in around difficult aspects of your childhood. Which allies arrive to support you with this? How do they support you?

I followed a path of lavender to the iron gate of my womb garden. I had to remove my armor to go in. When I entered, air blew the smells of flowers: roses, lavender, as well as the songs of birds. I saw owl, crow, bluebirds & hummingbirds.

I floated to the top of a tree where I was high above the garden, facing up and out towards the sky. This was being in my voice, my full expression, in a time of childhood where it didn't seem ok to be in my truth.

The meditation led me to an event where this was suppressed, and surprisingly, it was a time I was shopping with my mother for clothes as a teenager. I put on a skirt and she told me I looked like a hooker. I don't know exactly why that bothered me so much, or why it comes up in this context, but I was very offended. Although she was commenting on the skirt, I thought it was a judgement about me.

What would I say differently to this girl now? I think the badly conveyed intention here from my mother was: I want to protect you.

The irony is that if I had felt protected (loved and wanted), I may not have been interested in getting attention through sexy clothes. What I was missing there was feeling truly understood. That was the healing I brought to the girl in the dressing room. It connects to the voice, the expression of air, to be understood and then accepted for the way in which I wanted to express myself. Thalia

Imagine that there are beneficial herbal and flower allies in your Womb Garden that can teach you how to make medicinal preparations to support your emotional healing journey. Write out a conversation you have with each of these plant allies.

Imagine that you meet an ally in your Womb Garden who is your inner Wise One and carries all of the wisdom of your ancestral lineages about the beneficial use of herbs and flowers for emotional healing. Write out a conversation you might have with them, asking them any questions you might have about this and what their answers might be.

Imagine asking your inner Wise One about what kind of support you might want to enlist with professional herbalists, books, and/or research to support you in your explorations with medicinal herbs. Write out how they answer this question.

This week I was led by an indigenous woman who asked me to forgive my absentee father. I was guided to repeat his name 9 times, saying I forgive you for leaving.

I was also called upon to forgive my mother for not choosing a partner who would love and honor her this lifetime.

I was asked to reclaim my own destiny, that I can create my own relationships based on what is right for me, not preconditioned programming.

I was able to walk through this garden and feel supported by the abundance of trees and energy of renewal. I saw water and was called to it. Waterfalls appeared and I submerged myself in them, this seemed to be a process of letting go. Rebirth through water.

I see clearly that in previous relationships, my life experiences were suppressed. Although, some partners may have cared, I suppressed myself, which I never realized. All of my qualities and true calling in life was overlooked by many and I naturally diminished who I am for a relationship. I feel this will change who I allow into my life. I feel like a child, that I have not allowed myself to all of who I am in a relationship. I provided support to those who would never truly see me for who I am. Moon Star

Imagine that you visit your Womb Garden and the element of Earth has some gifts and wisdom for you and your inner child. What age does your inner child present as to receive the gifts of Earth? Are there any particular memories from your childhood that come up to receive these gifts?

I was supported by Baba Jaga during the meditation and was about 6 or 7 years old. I felt abandonment and the hurt feeling of being left by my parents when I was that age and sent to a tennis boarding school. This feeling of abandonment was opened to heal with the help of Baba Jaga and her big cauldron. I put this past hurt into the cauldron and it transformed into abundant love.

Baba Jaga showed me how to transform abandonment into unconditional love and my power animal raven gave me the following message: Like a bird, I can see my being from distance with observer eyes and let myself be filled with wisdom and freedom. I will continue listening to the Womb Garden or Womb Listening Meditation and also the Huul meditation that I regularly do to connect with Frau Holle and the Wyrding meditation to connect with the Womb of all Existence. That way I can rest and root within my own center and give myself all the healing that I need. Erika

Describe the gifts and wisdom the element of Earth has to offer you and your inner child. What beneficial effects do these gifts have for you, your inner child, and your life?

My Earth element allies were the pine trees that flanked the path to my Womb Garden. My father planted those trees. And once I entered the gates, I was in a forest of them, but there was no brush and only soft pine needles and cones on the earth beneath my feet. I could smell the pine and saw my inner child joyously looking down from her tree house that her father made.

Also, I had a very sweet memory of my aunt Nigh. My mother's sister's real name was Ellen, but I called her Nigh. She was a highly educated theologian and actually helped me survive the insanity of my home life, really as much as the land in Wisconsin. The memory was of she and I swinging on a swing my father had made between two giant pine trees. After a while the swing broke and we went boom on the tree roots beneath us. But we just laughed and laughed because neither of us was hurt. Shaun

Describe any memories you have of learning how to take care of your own physical needs growing up. Describe memories you have about the feelings your parents and other influential adults had about taking care of your physical needs for you and any feelings this brought up for you. (Food, clothing, housing, money...)

How do you feel these childhood experiences described in the previous questions influenced your abilities to take on adult responsibilities of caring for your own physical needs?

Describe any healing the Earth element and other allies you imagine have to offer you in your Womb Garden around these memories of getting your physical needs met. Are there any practical actions you can take in your life now to continue and nourish this healing process?

I called upon all my well ancestors and saw so many of them and also universal pre patriarchal figures showed up. There were also ancestors of a boyfriend I was really close to, there was aloe vera and cougar and the energy of smoky quartz. The diamond grid of the Earth was within my womb too and the smoky quartz was purifying and making crystalline my womb structure.

There was a warm feeling in my heart and groin. It felt like this was something to do with the fire element. We all went to the womb garden; I was seeing myself as the cougar and then I became the cougar. The gate of bones now had a few green creepers on them, one by one ancestral guardians of the womb garden appeared, I touched their feet and said I have come for more healing.

When asked to meet the wisest part of myself I reached a sacred sanctuary I had created a few years ago when I got started on the path, it's a white sand ocean with stone spiral and blue waters. There is an old woman with long white hair with white clothes there. We all wear white clothes only. She smiles at me saying that finally I've taken the time to come. I feel like telling her (maybe i do tell her through my feeling) that I have waited to come here again and am happy to be here (feels like a wisdom council of the Earth healing I am part of).

She energetically transmits that my image and energy on social media is an old self of mine and not attuned to my new energy body and I am connecting to old collective energy when I write or post. She asks me to take a break from there and then write from the womb a few months later.

We both look at the ages I needed the Earth energies more, it was when I was a month old in a crib always wanting to leave the body with my mum, when I was 3 years old, washing clothes alone at night, when I was 5 years old and met with an accident while crossing the road, and when I wanted to learn dance so badly. Dr. Sneha Rooh

I immediately felt at home with this journey, realizing from the outset how surprisingly connected I have always been with the earth element. For a long time in my teens and early adulthood I was so outside of myself that I had forgotten how deep rooted my earth connection is. The advantage of this is that I do not take it for granted and I nourish it regularly and celebrate and appreciate it deeply.

As a young infant I realize now that I had great difficulty maintaining, or perhaps ever establishing, my own boundaries. I was projected onto a lot by others in my family and I absorbed a lot of my family pain.

I am lucky to have had such an innate connection to nature that it has always protected me and supported me so even when I felt disconnected, unearthed, I have been able to trust in the nature of everything anyway. This has brought clarity about why I am so 'lucky', trusting and always have a sense of being protected and connected even at the most difficult of times. I gained the wisdom that at the age of 8 I became quite overwhelmed by my lack of boundaries, by others' emotions, strains, patterns, drama, projections, pain, that I lost myself, my joy, my bodily comfort.

I became quite outside of myself, quite sad in my outer world yet still trusting and somehow joyful in my inner world. Because I had nature anyway.

A fox led me from my garden gate to a mountain. I realize now the fox was a guide from my inner wise woman/hag, but it's funny because I had many nightmares about foxes as a girl. I wish I had received some guidance on these symbols then. But it's okay because I have had such a beautiful relationship with nature anyway. I have long since made friends with fox anyway. And I realize now that at age 8 I gained the wisdom of trust in nature by indeed losing myself. I'm grateful for this life lesson. It has served me well.

I joyfully thanked my 8-year-old self and gave her back her childhood sense of joy within her own body so she could feel whole and playful without the burden of everyone else's troubles. I explained to her that she need not carry any of this. She can be free to play and enjoy. Such a beautiful re-mothering moment to remove that burden from my little self.

I feel so much more able to move forward into revisiting the adolescent years that I had been feeling apprehensive of now. Because I am so much more whole. Donna-Lee Ida

Describe any strengths and skills around getting your physical needs met you learned from the childhood experiences described in the previous questions that you still benefit from today. Are there any ways you can nourish these strengths and skills to grow even more?

Take a moment to revisit a recent situation in which you had a big emotional reaction. Take some deep breaths and bring up the memory of that situation in as much detail as you can and the intensity of your emotional response. Now place your hands on your womb space and activate your Wise Womb Sanctuary. Imagine that your womb center has something called Placental Power that can easily distinguish between what belongs to the parent and what belongs to the child. Activate this Placental Power in your womb center and ask your Womb Wisdom what percentage of your recent emotional reaction belonged to your parent(s) and the emotional patterns you are still carrying for them and what percentage actually belongs to you in this current circumstance. Write down the percentages here:

- Belongs to my parent(s):

- Belongs to me in this current circumstance:

Now ask your Placental Power to activate and separate out the percentage that belongs to your parent(s) and remove it from your body. Take some deep breaths and allow yourself to make any sounds and/or body movements that feel supportive to this process. Once you feel complete, describe your experience with this here:

I can really feel that most of it was from my parents as I have noticed a shift every time I left the house or wasn't around them. 80 Percent comes up for the things from my parents.

Shaking it off, breathing with sound, delicious chocolate - anything that feels sensual! Writing down re-affirming things for myself and speaking them out loud with clear intent. (I did that as a candle spell and it feels great). Just relaxing and releasing the tension that builds in my belly sometimes to having to be or do this or that. Journaling. Burning some written words about it, maybe even creating a representation that can be burned, visualizing healthy boundaries for my parents in relation to me. Anna Rose

Please describe any circumstances in your life that are arising to offer you the opportunity to put what you are learning and shifting on this journaling journey into effect. Have you been able to respond to any relational behavior patterns in healthier ways? Are others responding to you differently? Does the overall energy of your life feel different in any way?

Coming of Age

Please share about any preparation you received prior to developing into your full adulthood around starting menstrual cycles, fertility, and sexuality. What education did you receive about it? From whom? What feelings were they having about sharing this with you? How did you feel receiving this information from them?

Please share about how the preparations for menstruation, fertility, and sexuality described in the previous question created a blueprint for your relationship with your womb and your adulthood. What belief systems did you adopt about it from the adults that were guiding you at this time?

If menstruation has been part of your womb journey, please write about any memories you have about your Menarche, your first menstrual cycle. How old were you? Do you remember seeing your blood for the first time? Any feelings you had about this? Who supported you? How did they support you? How did you feel about the support you received?

Please write about any memories you have about the first menstruation of other young people in your life when you were coming of age. Were you aware of anyone close to you starting to menstruate as you were coming of age? What how did their experiences influence yours?

Please share about your earliest sexual explorations with yourself and with others. When did you start self-pleasuring? What feelings did you have about this? When did you have your first kiss? How did this feel? Your first experiences with sensual touch?

Please share about how you felt about becoming an adult. Did you have any dreams or fantasies about what this meant for you? Did you have any awakening feelings of passion, desire, inner power? Did you have any dreams about who you would become as an adult? Were there any feelings that were uniquely your own, independent of the influences of others?

I felt like I was going to be in trouble when I became a woman. Life would be hard and unpredictable. I did not know how to deal with what was happening or what was supposed to happen. I imagined I would be like Lucy in Peanuts. Speaking her truth, strong, wise, and helping others. I thought I would be a great story teller and famous for these stories, nature, and helping others. These were more of my own from somewhere deep down, but also the women in my mother's side of the family were strong outspoken and incredibly infused with "magic powers" and intuition. I'd own a farm, take care of animals and keep nature pure and protected.
Jennifer

Please share about how your parents felt about you becoming an adult, your Menarche, fertility, and first sexual explorations. Did they have any fears about your development as a adult? Did they attempt to exert control over your behavior in any way? Did they offer you any support around any aspects of this challenging time of change?

What religious beliefs about gender, fertility, and sexuality were you raised with and encouraged to uphold as you grew into adulthood? Were there any beliefs about self-pleasuring that you struggled with? Were there any beliefs about sensual and sexual exploration outside of marriage that were compelling or difficult for you? Were there any beliefs about menstruation that influenced how you felt about this?

Please share about how your dreams, developing individual identity, and purpose in life were nurtured, supported, and encouraged. Or perhaps how they were neglected, suppressed, and discouraged.

Take a moment to ask your womb how much of your feelings about yourself at this time actually belonged to your parents and how much belonged to you. What percentages does your womb respond with? Ask your womb for guidance about any movement, breathing, sounding, and/or herbal ceremony practices you might do to give your parents feelings back to them so you can be free to simply feel your own feelings about this important time of your life. What does your womb offer you for this?

Please describe your relationship with your parents at the time that you started your first menstrual cycle.

How did your parents support you with your coming of age? How did they guide you in navigating menstruation and your budding sexuality/fertility?

Were there any other older mentors in your life at the time of your first menstruation that supported you in any way? If so, who were they and how did they support you?

Were there any tensions between you and your parents at the time of your first menstruation? If so, please describe.

What were your parents' feelings, attitudes, and practices around menstruation like? Do you have any memories of interactions about this that you had with them during your childhood? What did you learn or adopt for yourself from these experiences?

What were the feelings and attitudes of the other adult menstruators in your life about menstruation throughout your childhood? What memories do you have about other menstruators besides your parent sharing about this? What did you learn or adopt for yourself from these experiences?

Do you have any memories of how your parents related to each other about menstruation? What did you learn or adopt for yourself from this awareness?

How did your parents approach sexuality in your home growing up? Did you ever experience their sexuality together in any way? If so, please describe. How did this experience influence the development of your sexuality?

Did your parents ever talk with you about masturbation? If so, what did they say and how did it influence you?

Did your parents ever share with you about their feelings of life purpose, following spiritual guidance, and/or their passions and inspirations in life? If so, please describe. How did what they shared influence your experiences of this for yourself?

Do you remember your parents supporting your feelings of passionate purpose, inspiration, and/or vision for your life at this time of Menarche? Did they support your creative expression in any way? Please describe.

Do you remember having any feelings of passionate purpose, inspiration, and/or vision for your life at this time, supported or not? If so please describe and share what has become of those feelings and dreams as you have traveled through life.

If Divine Mother was guiding your parents in supporting you during your time of Menarche, preparing you when you were younger, and guiding you through this important initiation, what might they have done differently? What would you have liked to receive from your parents?

I would have received more love, understanding, and nurturing during my formative years. I would have been given ceremony for shedding blood. I would have been held, loved and supported, as my body changed. I would have received a journal. My mother would have told me I am powerful and I am safe. My mother would have shown me kindness and not embarrass me in front of family members. My mother, if she were guided by Divine Mother, would have given me rose quartz. Moon Star

I would have loved to receive a rites of passage ceremony. I would have loved to learn about the blood mysteries and how it meant that I was powerful and magical. I would have loved to be with other women and girls of all ages to hold space for me and to help me feel more comfortable in my skin and more accepting of what was to come. Willow

Unconditional love and wisdom is what I could have liked to receive. She would have given me the science and spiritual part of the cycles. The cosmic part. Wow, there's just so much. However, what I have done for myself over the past few years is exactly what I would have liked to receive from my mother. Jennifer

Examples of loving relationship and an understanding of my own innocent pace of development. I'd have liked her to be more whole so she could have demonstrated that to me. Donna-Lee Ida

Take a moment to listen to your Womb Wisdom and ask what it might look like to do a Coming-of-Age Menarche Celebration Ceremony for yourself retroactively. What guidance does your womb offer you for this? How would you have liked to have been celebrated and initiated? How can you do this for yourself now?

Stillness, wise, acceptance, allow new people who can guide you enter into your life. Allow new people to enter your life. Allow new people to enter your life. Moon Star

Writing a letter to myself at the Menarche stage telling everything and describing in detail what I needed but didn't receive back then. Keeping this letter as form of missing piece to reweave myself back into wholeness. Also doing a ritual and ceremony for myself to welcome and celebrate my menstruation blood.

Slavic Goddess Mokosh was present and I felt the urge to call an online co-creative circle where I finished embroidering the Goddess Mokosh on my menstruation panties and did a meditation to call her in. The Goddess Mokosh was very present throughout the whole Menarche phase. She stands for weaving of fate, Motherhood and protection of Mother Earth.

I have reconnected even stronger with the Fate Weaver Mokosh, the three Norns and have realized how my creativity and handcrafts are part of my life purpose, also integrating and weaving new technologies as well as tradition into the new tapestry of humanity. Erika

Please share about any older adults who had already passed through menopause that were part of your life growing up and how they influenced you.

Please share about any Menopausal adults that were involved in your life when you were approaching Menarche. What influence did they have on you at this time?

Please share about any feelings you have about getting older. Do you have any practices aimed at diminishing the effects of again on your body? If so, what are they?

I love getting older, it is like falling in love with all my body parts and feelings more and more. Like my main Beregini and embroidered symbol in my dress which I connect with on many occasions during the day, I feel very much like the crone, the wise one. Much more so than the Menarche which I never was able to properly live out. I have my practices with the Runes, handcrafts, witchy ceremonies that connect me with my Crone wisdom. Erika

Do you have any fears or concerns about growing older? If so, please describe.

How did you feel about growing older when you were going through your Menarche? Did you have any fears or concerns then? How do the fears and concerns you had then relate to the fears and concerns you have now about growing older?

How were your fears and concerns about growing older when you were going through Menarche (first menstruation) effected by your experiences of menopausal adults at that time? How do those experiences relate to your current fears and concerns about growing older?

Take a few moments to connect with your inner Wise One and ask them for guidance about the process of growing older and how you might alleviate the fears of your young self as well as your current fears. What wisdom, strengths, and skills can you celebrate learning as you have grown older? Write about what they have to offer you.

Imagine your inner Wise One having a conversation with your young self as you were coming of age and beginning your menstrual journey. Write out that conversation, offering your young self the wisdom of your inner Wise One about the strengths and powers they will grow into as an adult. Include any questions your young self might have had and the answers your Wise One has for them.

I became aware during the ancestral council meeting of some of the supplies that want to be present. Berries, pomegranate seeds, beet juice or menstrual blood, dark chocolate, womb anointing oil, and rose tincture. The altar that was created by my well of womb ancestors Rose and Iguela looked like the sacred medicine wheel of the four directions. There were rose petals that outlined the entire circle. Each spoke was to hold space for each of the 4 lineages that I come from. There was a circle that surrounded this altar. All of the ancestors who I know and are in my memory were present. It was hard to be with two of my ancestors. One I could feel myself wanting to squirm away from, yet I stood there and held as much love as I could. My animal allies and herbal allies were present. I was anointed with oils on my womb and dried blood on my third eye in the shape of an upturned crescent moon. I was given a red hood and a fur coat to wear from Rose. Willow

Imagine you could go back in time and become the mentor for your young self that you would have loved to have and offer to organization a celebratory ceremony for your coming of age. Write out a conversation you would have with your young self, planning out the details of this celebration.

I feel more drawn to simple ink drawings again as a creative pastime I used to do a lot as a teen. I feel alive with creative fire and look forward to finding how this unfolds for me in my life work. I feel my hearts desires are becoming real again, I'm open to relationship again. I feel Venus is stirring hot within me for her renewed life after being healed of the adolescent trauma that made her a ghost previously. Donna-Lee Ida

I recently created two beautiful gardens in honor of my inner maiden. As often is this case...I didn't realize it until just now. It came instinctively, but I didn't realize how therapeutic it was going to be...I planted all my favorite flowers and am experimenting with using more space. I'm most excited about vine plants for some reason... pumpkin, squash, morning Glory, loofa, roses and anything that climbs. I also painted a lovely energetic piece where my inner feminine was fed through the roots by the masculine in honor of the full flower moon....

Lavender and peony's...

Crickets and birdsong...

Naked sun-soaked afternoons with a good book...

Planting more seeds than I can count...

Full with Spring....

Overflowing onto the earth.

Shaydden

Menarche with Inanna

By Jessica Huckabay

My 11-year-old self tells me how she wants to celebrate her Menarche

Eyes bright with wonder that someone is listening to her heart's desire

She asks me to set up the Red Tent amidst the wildflowers and edible weeds

We pull the screen tent out of the back of the van and the great red bag with the collection of red fabrics

Velvet, satin brocade, chiffon, varied shades from vixen red to deep burgundy wine

And her favorite, magenta

We drape the fabrics over mats that press down the knee-high grasses and pin them up on the walls of the tent

Creating a billowing patchwork of red

An artist's meditation on what this color can evoke

We make a circle of precious stones

Place a statue of Divine Mother I made out of clay in the center

We anoint our brows

The base of our skulls

Our hearts and wombs

With rose ointment

And go inside

We dance, sing songs, no words

Just painting the air with vowels spinning out from the womb

She asks me to spend the whole day in there

With her

The next time I bleed

And tell her stories of Innana's great boat of Heaven

How Innana's vulva

Could grow as large as a boat

For her to sail around on.

And how when Innana's grandfather Enke

Stole her powers once

Her powers to see in the dark

Awaken passion in the heart of her lover with the sound of her whisper

Hear the voices of plants

Usher babies into the world

And dying friends out of it

Peacefully

Her powers to transmit healing energy with her hands, breath, and voice

To heal herself with movement and sound

Her powers to weave webs of connection that surround the whole world

And cultivate mutually nurturing relationships with all beings

Her powers to understand the influence of the sun, moon, and stars on the flow of life here on Earth

To journey to the center of the Earth to replenish and rejuvenate

Her powers to recycle emotional energy back into pure vitality

And see into the soul of any lover, friend, or family member to discover the best ways to relate

Her powers to dance between intimacy and solitude with grace

And connect with her own inner wisdom to guide her through a life of peace and ease

She wants me to tell her what powers Enke couldn't steal

About the nameless, formless power underneath all the rest

That rises up through the Earth, showing our feet the way

And descends from the sky through the crown of our heads

Guiding our eyes to see the path forward

Our ears to hear the truth

Our mouths to speak that truth clearly

Our noses to smell out lies

Nobody can take these powers from anyone if they don't let them

Enke had to be tricky to steal the powers he did steal

But Innana is quite tricky too.

She arrived at his house with a delicious feast and great kegs of beer

With loving hands and a laughing voice, she fiested him into a drunken slumber

The she hummed a joyful tune as she gathered and stuffed all of her stolen powers

Into her vulva

Which swelled up to become the Boat of Heaven

And she sailed off down the river

When Enke awoke and discovered what had happened

He laughed at his foolishness

He sent his porters down the river after her but knew they would never be able to catch her

We sing more songs to celebrate this story

She tells me she wants to meet me in the Red Tent regularly

Hear more stories

Sing more songs

Watch this wildflower patch change through the seasons

And stuff our powers back into our vulvas

One by one

Until we too could sail off down the river

Too fast and clever for any old grandfather to catch us

Of course, my love, I tell her

That is exactly what we shall do

This Stone

By Jessica Huckabay

This stone has tasted river water only a few times in its centuries-long life on the surface of the Earth. For at one point, it was in the creek bed, where the waters flowed, bathing and smoothing it into the round flat shape it now holds. But there was one great flood hundreds of years ago that stretched out across this valley, dispersing this stone and all of its brothers and sisters into fractal villages to bake in the sun until the next flood calls them home.

This stone heard my murmurings of longing for the knowledge of where my placenta might be, Knowing my actual placenta, the sacred site of merging between my mother and I that fed me and taught me for 9 months, delivering my spirit into my physical body, and so wisely knew how to release me, giving me as a gift into the world, knowing this sacred web of wisdom was tossed into the medical waste bin in the hospital with no recognition of its continued power to connect me to a new mother, Mother Earth.

This stone heard my plans to create a substitute placenta with a stone, some of my hair, and some menstrual blood, and bury it in the ground under a rose bush.

This stone raised itself to the surface of the dry creek bed wildflower meadow bordering my herb garden, like raising its hand as a volunteer. It sat clear of any clinging dirt, exposed in a clear patch, letting the sun light up its perfect mass, its round and somewhat rough edges, and mottled grey brown and green stripes creating veins of Earth wisdom perfect to continue my education.

This stone did not need to preen or pose. Its perfection was so clear, there was no need to prove anything. It's contentment with its own presence was so well established, its confidence about being in the right place at the right time, its sentience so complete and connected with the whole of everything, that it awoke in me an instant knowing that this was the right rock substitute for my lost placenta.

Now this rock resides under the growing roots of a rose bush, seeping messages from my menstrual blood through the soil through root networks, veins of stone knowing, down to the core of Mother Earth, and delivers her wisdom and nourishment directly to my blood, through my navel, through my witch's 3rd eye at the base of my skull.

This stone provides transport to any part of my life in which I suffered from the lack of this connection, this nourishment, this wisdom.

This stone invites me to visit my Menarchal self and sing the veins of connection into being for her. It carries me underground, through the tunnels of moles and worms, through the hollow roots of dead trees, through the electro-chemical signal ways of mushrooms to the twelve-foot square patch of inner-city yard in San Francisco behind the flat where I lived on 7th Avenue and Irving in the Sunset district when I was 11 years old and got my first period.

This stone shows me how to transmit my energy and wisdom to all of the stones in that patch of yard, into the roots of the great Eucalyptus tree that stretched taller than the 5-story building we lived in, above the leaking roof, into the universal sky. This stone and I share the signature geometry of my blood with all of the living beings surrounding my young self. The tree, the stones, the bushes all sigh in relief, to finally be let in on the true nature of this new potency they had smelled, sensed, longed to connect with but had been deprived the taste of her first blood.

This stone radiates Earth Alchemy, meeting the longing of this living community to know me, transforming my pre-menopausal blood into the new blood it was then. Every stone, worm, weed, bush, leaf on that great tree, celebrates this return to reverence, this emergence of new life, this devotion that has carried me back to my unrecognized burgeoning self.

This stone and I gaze up as my 11-year-old self emerges out onto the balcony 5 stories up with a pomegranate. We wonder if she can feel our silent songs of joy, the whole yard dancing invisibly at her love of this primordial fruit. We wonder if she tastes the mythology in those plump red morsels of sweet tart exploding on her tongue. We wonder if she feels the future poems she will write as they gather in her belly like so many pomegranate seeds.

This stone and I smile with confidence that this young woman will find her way, that we can silently radiate our knowing of her worth through her pathways through this city and beyond, informing all of the trees of her presence, letting them know of her DNA structures, how to reach her with just the right rustle of leaves and gleam of rainbow bark. That everywhere she turns, she would feel a welcoming from the rocks, the soil, the green growing things, not just through the sharing of breath, but also the sharing of weight, feet carving pathways through space like roots spread wide, holding the swaying trunk and branches of her life as it grows.

This stone and I have delivered the gift of her sensations to the family of life to share.

Tongue prying pomegranate seeds loose from the white membrane

Cascade of seeds tumbling into her mouth

Sounds of city life rushing into her ears

Meeting the pulse of blood on the other side of her eardrums

Wind caressing her skin

Eyes following the sway of hanging branches

Following the drop of seed pods

Buttocks growing cold on the metal grate of the balcony floor

Opening movement in the belly by dropping legs over the edge

Feet and calves swinging from the knees

Intensity of focus on savoring every pip

Without breaking the membrane

Without leaking any juice out

Before it lands in her mouth

Each drop precious

Licking them off finger tips

Explosions of juice in the mouth

As teeth crush their round perfection

If it weren't for her, this stone would not feel that cascade of seeds, that explosion of juice, that preciousness.

If it weren't for her, the tree would never feel feet swinging over the edge, or buttocks growing cold.

Her presence, sharing the wind caressing her skin with all of the other skins in the yard, bark, stone faces, leaves green with chlorophyll, her eyes witnessing the dance of tree branches, offering a layering of sentience, turning life into a delicate pastry with rich crispness folded and flaking between the layers of cream.

Chapter Two: Creative Fertility, Partnership, Soul Purpose, and Wisdom

In this chapter we will explore the gifts of creativity, fertility, partnership, soul purpose, and wisdom as they show up through the lifecycle portals of our fertile years, our partnering and parenting journeys, our reclamation/re-alignment with our soul purpose during the perimenopausal phase/time frame, and the wisdom of the menopausal/wisdom years.

Creative Fertility

Please describe any strengths our gifts you are blessed with in your creative expression. Do you also feel you have similar strengths or gifts in your sexual expression?

I have a particular ability to draw, and people say I have a very distinctive and recognizable style. The way I think of it is that I see a beauty that comes from within, and that complements what I see on the outside. At least, I used to, though I lost so much of what came naturally to me, when I was ill, that I am still recovering my creative flow and my sense of myself as an artist.

I mostly work from imagination, working with images that are generated by my feelings and experience. I think I have a sensitivity for color, and am slowly learning oil painting in order to explore more deeply the subtleties of color.

This is such an interesting question and I'm looking for connections. I suppose I do have a sensitivity for touch, subtlety and nuance. I have been pretty much single for about 15 years, but I used to have a lot of imaginative and spiritual experiences during sex, would see lovers turn in to animals, and basically go on journeys. My body sensations would make my body feel distorted or dissolving, drifting in a sea or into the cosmos, in fact it might be simpler to say I find it hard to stay in normal reality during sex. Pennifer Moonmama

I am blessed with handcrafts and embroidery in particular. I have never felt more empowered than when I embroidered my destiny towel "Rushnyk", my destiny dress or the womb pouch with 27 Beregini (Goddesses) symbols. I also love to paint and dance freely and wildly. I always feel my Shakti energy flowing really freely and wildly and I feel full of power and beauty like the Red Tara or Karakulla like she is also known. I feel seductive and joygasmic when I dance or connect with certain Beregini symbols like the Muse or Creatrix for example. Erika

Please describe any challenges or limitations you feel you have in your creative expression. Do you feel you have correlating challenges or limitations in your sexual expression?

Please share about how your creative expression and sexual expression is or has been influenced by your menstrual cycle and/or your relationship with lunar cycles and seasonal changes.

I remember discovering that the premenstrual phase, particularly the night before I began menstruating was a very powerful time creatively and psychologically. I would stay up late making my most powerful art work, or at least the most powerful ideas, sketches, and insights. It all goes together. Art is about the process rather than a production, and I often wished I could tap deeper into this source on a more regular basis. I would also have longer cycles of being intensely interested in expressing something through creativity, and then needing to focus in other directions for some time. Pennifer Moonmama

It is like free-flowing Kundalini energy and directly connected to each other. If I tend to my sexuality, my creativity flows like a river, and if it doesn't then I find it hard to be creative. Erika

When I really think about it -my sexual energy is expressed in subtly different ways than my creative energy. My sexuality feels deeper and more grounded towards my root center- while my creativity is definitely higher and more whimsical and flowy... However, expressing my sexuality in a creative way can be a wonderful mesh of the two.

I tend to be creative or sexual in waves...

However, I've only began to explore the schedule and Dynamics of it the last couple years or so.... it's really dependent on how I regulate my overall energy first and foremost. The way I treat my body on a daily basis.

I feel surging sexual energy when ovulating. When I don't actually have sex during this time...my body will cycle the energy and it feels very orgasmic. Often times jolting me with orgasm even at work or wherever lol ... I've been exploring with this for a couple years now... My creative energy is felt strongly generally closer to menstruation where I feel more deeply centered as a conduit between worlds...I often make time to let things move thru me during this time. In both cases I believe I'm touching into the divine...in subtly different ways... Shaydden

Excerpts of Jessica Huckabay's writings...

As a result of watching my mother abused, invalidated, and exploited throughout my childhood was that I had no great desire to get married have children myself. I was also quite averse to intimacy with a lover as I projected my fears about getting into an abusive relationship with a man onto them. As soon as I caught one whiff of something that resembled my step father's behavior, I would withdraw into myself. My womb would recoil all of my sexual desire. I had several relationships in a row that suffered the slow death this produced. I longed for intimacy, connection, to be close to someone who would be there for me and whom I could love. But I didn't know anything about what that looked or felt like. And as soon as I became sexually intimate with someone and the initial infatuation wore off after 3 months, I would start judging them for all of the ways they resembled my father.

It is difficult for men to not resemble my father as they were raised by men just like my father who passed down generations of trauma and unhealthy patterns of masculine identity that taught them to soothe their wounds and nourish themselves by feeding off of women. The hierarchy of patriarchy convinces them that the higher up on the tower they can get, the happier they will be. The more people they exploit and step on, the few will be above them doing the same to them. This tower of masculinity has no place for women, except as the trophy wives of the men at the top of the tower and the soothers of those lower down who are getting stepped on. For many men, stepping on their women is the easiest way to get a leg up, because other men will fight for their own position. Women have been groomed in this system to soothe and appease.

Often, I found myself with no available ways of expressing myself sexually except with myself. As I have a great deal of it to express, and a lot of feelings about all aspects of this, I quickly discovered that I could express it through creativity. Writing poetry, making artwork, and applying my creative inspiration to crafting a life that avoided many of the entrapments of society.

My longing for sexual fulfillment compelled me to initiate myself into creative fertility. I sat in front of my altar in the tiny converted water tower I was living in. I was approaching the rocky bottom of my barrel, felt alone and in despair. My last romantic relationship had landed in the same dehydrated soup packet of celibate monogamy as the one prior to that one and I had moved away as my career aspirations where we had been living together had also dried up. So, in the dark, slanted water tower I sat, facing my altar, calling out to Kali, the goddess of transformation, and that's when I felt it. A pillar of creative energy rising up from my womb through my core. I could inhale and draw it up until it poured out into my hands and mouth. I knew this energy was my creative fertility. It was a gift from my womb.

This was not the first time this energy had flowed for me. I had been writing poetry and making artwork with this energy for over a decade, but this time I was consciously aware of where this energy was coming from. I had made a decision in that moment to devote my creative fertility to my artistic creations.

I still longed for an intimate partner, however. It seemed important to fulfill this desire in a new and different way. This longing for partnership has been strong in my lineage, and all of the unfulfilled desires of my ancestors had built up inside me to create a steady determination. Every time a relationship would crumble, I would cry out to the Goddess, pleading with her to tell me why this one didn't develop into the closeness and intimacy I was longing for. I begged her to show me what I needed to do to find the one that I would be able to build this with. Her answer was always the same.

"Focus on loving yourself, your inner healing work. When you are ready, your partner will be there."

It seems this activation of my creative fertility was an important part of this inner healing work. My fertility cycle was guiding me towards creative endeavors that prepared me for fulfilling my soul purpose. This was primary. Only when that journey was ready for me to have a partner was I able to join with one.

Please describe any painful symptoms you experience during your menstrual cycle/fertility/sexuality and any ways you see these symptoms as symbolic of the challenges and limitations you feel in your creative expression.

Do you notice certain times in your menstrual cycle, the lunar cycle, and/or the seasonal cycles when you feel more inclined to be creative? Less inclined? More inclined to create and share outwardly? More inclined to create just for yourself? Please describe.

Were there any times in your past when your creativity was discouraged or suppressed that you feel to bring healing to? Imagine you could go back and visit your younger self who was experiencing this and support them in some way. Write a story about this visit and describe the healing process.

Please share about any creative fertility practices that you have explored from your own inspiration. Include stories about your exploration of creative writing, art, dance, music, crafting, sewing, interior decorating, gardening, etc.

Please share about anything that is limiting or diminishing your creative fertility at this time and which of these practices feel like they might help to get it flowing again.

What creative practices might you like to implement in your life regularly to nourish and develop your creative fertility? What strategies might you implement to prioritize these practices?

I became much more attune to the smells that I smelled outside and how they made me feel. I noticed that I was also appreciating these smells for gracing my nose and stimulating my senses. This brought me joy and felt like I had a secret with myself. I have begun making mental notes regarding which smells I am smelling and what I think it means to me. I am so happy to have reconnected in this way with herbs.

I am also currently collaging all of these trinkets and old gizmos in my room onto a wooden post. It is messy, cute, complex, and gooey pot of art stew. It reminds me of everything swimming in my womb. The process is slow, but I am slowly decluttering my room and stringing together meaning through the process. I feel motivated to organize the piles of trinkets waiting to be stuck in a new spot, which brings me hope that my womb wants s to meaning-make, be organized and listened to. Ava

Excerpts from Jessica Huckabay's writings...

What these men didn't know I hungered for was a different kind of touch than they were offering, a touch that gave more than it took, a touch of reverence and recognition of my power. I longed for a touch that saw me on the inside, heard my poetry, all aspects of it, including the parts that cut deep gashes in the swollen gangrene of the wounded feet of society, willing to amputate, if necessary, to drain us of our pain as well as the parts that delighted in the sensual pleasures of life. I wanted a touch that listened to my voice and gave it value and was willing to transform itself to become new with me. I wanted to be touched by someone that could receive the depth of my claws, scraping through the masks to the core of the person, revealing their vulnerable greenness, the newness we all share in the face of the unknown. I wanted to be touched by someone who had the capacity to consider my feelings, needs, and desires equally to their own. It was clear to me that these men offered none of these touches. And even if they did, I was too busy developing my own ability to receive these touches, to even know what I was longing for, that I could not see it in them.

It was clear to me in that moment on the bench, looking out over the verdant valley, that in order to create the life I was meant to have, I must listen to these moments of silent connection, taking in all of the nourishment available in the air, the blue of the sky, the moisture of the clouds, the heat of the sun radiating through the green photosynthesizing leaves, releasing molecules of medicine, morsels of pleasure straight to my nose, heart, brain, limbs, caressing the hairs on my arms and legs to erect stances of attention and swirling sways of delight. I knew that in order to create anything big, like the fulfilling life I longed for in a world bent on reserving this privilege for a very small few, sick with greed for luxury and willing to lie, cheat, steal, murder to fill their infinite emptiness, I must evoke the most potent power from within, a power that was the opposite greed and taking and domination. I knew this power resided in the pulsing of life that could not be suppressed completely no matter how much cement was spread across the surface of the earth, there would still be this power pressing up through the cracks in sharp unstoppable green shoots of grass. I knew this power was generously tucked away in every seed of every plant, every egg of every insect, fish, bird, reptile, and in every ovary, testicle, womb of every mammal. I knew this power to create started with the burst of orgasmic pleasure we were all wired to desire and seek. Many have attempted to harness this power for personal gain and seem to succeed, seducing the hungry masses with lies about its nature, disrupting our instincts with shame, severing this fertility from its true source, the uprising of life from the core of the planet, pulsing through our feet in collectively celebrated reverence for Mother Earth. But I knew that harnessing it would only backfire, especially for me, for my mission compelled me to adhere to ancestral contracts, living out the answers to thousands of lifetimes burdened with unfulfilled prayers, the weight of which would crush me into a smear of depressive oblivion if I strayed one centimeter from the living path of truth I was sworn to serve.

Before I was born sworn.

I knew I had to let this power take me through its paces, leading me through obstacle courses of repeating unsatisfactory relationship patterns to recognize that blaming others just kept me from ever connecting with this power. For its left foot stands on a bedrock of self-responsibility that is deeper than roots, molten at the bottom so close it gets to the source of life in the womb of Gaia.

I knew I had to learn to breath and feel all of my desire, sorting through the lies, sifting out the gems, the seeds.

I learned I could plant those seeds in my own womb, leave them in the dark, and water them with my tears, my solitude, my compassion, my longing. They gestated there for many years through the coldness of delusions, until the heat of this late spring finds them sprouting through my rich grey hair. Finally, I can breathe fully, after burning away the obstructions with countless hours of pranayama and asana practice, observing the yamas and niyamas, polishing this flower pot vessel for this life of longing for this final blossoming of desire. Now I know that the grand images I once had of the colors and aromas this bloom would finally offer could not live up to the deeply rooted satisfaction of this cracked pot with soil spilling back to the garden floor, roots winding through the cracks with worms and microbes, and stems reaching out from under the shadows of the past, reaching from the sun, finally bursting open swollen buds to the tickling hairy feet of bees.

Partnership

Please share about qualities you nurture in yourself to foster healthy partnerships in your life.

Flow, don't be afraid of your depth and beauty. Let it show. Nurture expressions of feeling. Be gentle and kind and patient.

Calmness, patience, a capacity for holding space around discomfort. A strength of spirit that need not diminish flow/expression. Gentle strength and active attention. Donna-Lee Ida

Love, compassion, nurturance, gentleness, the ability to rest and receive, flow

Hold space for my feelings to move through, protection and reassurance of my inner child, inner support if I'm feeling a lack of confidence. Aggie

The qualities I nurture in myself to foster healthy partnership is honesty about where I am, communication of what's happening in the moment, forgiveness and understanding. Room to grow, balance, and structure.

Manifestation, creation, cycles, endings and new beginnings. Plan and prepare.

Knowing the season and its energy. The elements and energy of the earth, cosmos, body, blood, existence, time and love working with them. Jennifer

I practice gratitude every day and write gratitude messages to my community for the past two years. That has helped me to go to bed with an open and grateful heart and eyes for even the smallest nice things in my life. I can so connect more and more with people from the heart and build deep and trustworthy relationships. I also love my creative and outgoing nature that I practice through my embroidery practices and also through dancing and regular chats with good friends.

I love to dance, tell wise stories, paint and embroider, jade egg exercises and sexuality in general. I have the qualities of the Red Tara and Baba Yaga, all wild and also highly sensual.

I have discipline to do my morning practices of shamanic movements to connect with my seven Bereginis/Goddesses, practicing yoga regularly and resilience to stay on the path while also feeding myself with good books and things to learn on an ongoing basis. Erika

The quality of being able to hold space for myself, in my emotions and triggers. I am trying to nurture a healthy sense of boundaries for myself and others. The ability to discern what is my wounds reacting and what needs I have, if they come from a genuine place or a place where I need to give it to myself. Creating a safe and compassionate space for myself and others. Patience is a hard one but still. I think most important is the willingness and commitment to own growth, caretaking and healing.

A great mothering to soothe myself and hold myself in my emotions. A great portal to open my heart with myself and to feel inspired in hard moments. Strong messages about what I need or what is right through my body. A deep sense of connection that is felt with myself but also with guides and ancestors and Mother Earth. A connection to the bigger picture.

A strength that protects, brings me back to focus, gives me a discipline that is needed to come closer to myself and healthier ways of being, feeling seen in myself, a strong will in pursuing my dreams and what I feel is right to do, a sense of structure. Anna Rose

Please share about any imbalanced or unhealthy patterns you have noticed in yourself around partnership, either from the past or currently. How are you endeavoring to bring these patterns into greater balance?

Describe what qualities a domination-based relationship has and what qualities a partnership relationship has.

Which domination-oriented qualities do you notice in your relationship with yourself? With others?

What qualities does your Divine Self have to offer in your partnership with yourself?

How can you come into greater integrity with these divine qualities that support you to have healthy partnerships with self and other and express them more in how you live your life?

When you reflect on the primary relationships you have with people in your life, which ones feel like they nurture you as much or more than you nurture them?

If there are any primary relationships that don't feel balanced in how they nurture you compared to how you nurture them, in what ways do they nurture you that you can cultivate more appreciation for?

As you focus on gratitude and appreciation for the ways you are being nurtured and cared for, what changes in the feeling of energetic balance between you?

What can you ask for in any of your relationships that feel imbalanced that would help to right that balance?

Are there any secret agreements that you can bring into the light of awareness that are perpetuating any imbalances in your relationships? How can you revise these agreements and make them explicit and openly agreed upon?

What kind of partnership agreements would you like to grow into in your life?

What are some ways you can move towards more partnership-oriented relationships and release any domination-oriented patterns in your relationships?

Please share about any imbalances, frictions, or turbulence you have felt between your inner polarities, ie: masculine/feminine energies, dark/light, active/inactive, pain/pleasure, etc. Are any of these polarities in a domination relationship with their polar partners?

Please share about practical ways these polarized energies show up in your life. How do your inner polarities effect your relationships? How do they reflect the frictions in those relationships? How do they reflect the harmony?

How do the domination patterns in your inner polarities show up in your relationships?

Please describe some practical ways you can care for the frictions in your relationships and nurture harmony.

I made a commitment to myself to honor the need to express my feelings without feeling the need to put a lid on myself...and with loving compassion toward myself about expressing my true feelings without shame or fear of being too much will help me to better navigate choices of who and how I engage in relationships. Donna-Lee Ida

I consciously take time out when I am bleeding, meeting in women's circles, dance and express myself creatively like through sacred embroidery or womb art or womb dance. I can also nurture myself with good herbs in support of my cycles. Erika

How might you shift towards partnership relationships between your inner polarities? How might this effect your relationships with others?

Please share your vision for the kinds of co-creative partnerships you would like to nourish in your life. What feelings and qualities do you want them to have? What feelings and qualities do you want them to be free of?

Relationships where I can express/ask for something I prefer or desire and feel pleasure about receiving it. I also am able to honor this for other people. I imagine my relationships where communication comes from a space of self-awareness and security with whatever comes up. Language is more positive and less defensive. There is mutual respect. I want them to be free of positioning to be bigger, better, deeper, or higher. There is a mutual respect for each other's talents and areas of challenge. Honesty and abilities to make mistakes while owning it versus trying to pound the other person down. Free of guilt language. Free of putting oneself down.
Jennifer

I like to nourish more co-creative relationships where we practice honest and non-violent communication, where we aim to grow together and have the willingness for ongoing learning and support. I like to experience the feelings of trust, integrity and sovereignty. And I want them to be free from judgement, free from unwillingness to be open to learn new things. Erika

Please share about any practical skills you feel you need to learn to nurture co-creative partnerships in your life. Please share some practical steps you can take towards developing these skills including any support you might need to set up for yourself to do so.

I need to learn to revisit non-violent speaking and compassion. I need to learn how to develop sharper skills dealing with guilt. I need to allow myself to feel good in areas I didn't before. I need to repair parts of relationships where I was dominant. I need to feel okay about feeling okay. I need to soothe myself when I get nervous. I need to slow down a little more especially when I feel myself sped up. Jennifer

Forgiveness and humor, plus ongoing communication skills. Erika

Soul Purpose Alignment

Imagine you have an inner wisdom guide that is helping you to align with your soul purpose. This guide shows up in the form of menstrual symptoms and/or other health challenges as well as life circumstances that may seem like obstacles, but if you listen to your wisdom guide, you start to understand how everything is conspiring towards your soul purpose fulfillment. Write about what this wisdom guide might look like if they were a person in as much detail as possible.

She is strong, active and fearless, but soft and loving, and acts with kindness. She is beautiful and has a rose light about her. She also has something of gold in her nature. She seems to me to be related to the maiden, like a mirror image of maiden energy.

She carries a pot, in which she has kept safe all the treasures of my adolescence that might have got lost or broken along the way if she hadn't been caretaking them for me. She is fearless in and with love; she is strong enough to love. I trust her.

In my body she is a huge snake, with a heavy, grounded feeling, very earthed. She carries the original life force energies, plus a knowing that comes from lived experience. She is accepting of death and taking responsibility for her life. She is moving in a slow, smooth figure eight movement in my hips. I recognize her as the origin of my inner rhythms. Pennifer Moonmama

The Red Tara or Karakulla appeared, offering me joygasmic vitality and the awakened snake of life force energy and limitless creativity. She told me that it is absolutely fine to use my sexuality as a driving force without inhibition. I do not need a partner to feel my boundless creativity and joygasmic flow. I just need to center myself on my sacral power and act from my essence there. Erika

My Enchantress came to me in a meadow full of flowers and herbs. She was wearing a white flowing dress and had long white hair plaited down her back. She had a cauldron in front her, a cosmic cauldron of time. She told me I had 'passed the test'. I also received a message from her about working more with voice. She brought me the gift of deeper realizations of certain significant events that have been woven through my last several perimenopause years, and of my menopausal Rite of Passage that my Bio Mystical Womb Healing Journey so magically aligned with, and was to became my Rite of Passage into my Wise Woman phase of my life. The wisdom she offered unfolded over the next several weeks.

The following weeks after I met with my Enchantress my connection with nature expanded as the voice of nature came flooding with clarity, into my awareness. A story of the the Ancestors began to unfold from the Brambles, the blackberry bushes that surround my garden, and from those that live down the lane from me. They were telling me what they had witnessed over time. How the Ancestors connected with them and how to pick of their fruits so there were plenty for all creatures to share. I listened as they told me blood stories and how the remembering is stored within them. The living library. The Enchantress was showing up for me before this Bio Mystical Womb Journey in different ways. The test she told me I had passed in the opening ceremony was the promise I had made to myself 5 years previous that I was ready to commit time to myself, my own needs, and my work as Shamanic therapist. Over those years as my relationships with others that were draining for me finished, the Enchantress began showing in me again in the empowerment in being able to live on my own, being comfortable in my own company, with my animal plant and stone friends, connecting with nature, and also being able to show up for family and close friends. The voice she spoke of in the ceremony became the voice of nature and the voice of womb. Listening to both voices. and both voices being One. Hazel

I felt the enchantress as the muse, as the goddess of love and as the primal goddess all together in one energy. She first came through as Mary Magdalene at the opening and wanted to be sung through me as the chant "Kundalini Mata Shakti Mata Shakti Namo Namo." As we danced, she moved through me softly, sweetly and gave me gentle invitations to pull my attention to my senses and to being ever-present in my body. I experienced her as intimate, as a sensual embodied awareness. She asked me to be ever-present, and to feel each caress, each move, each feeling as sacred, captivating and all-consuming. She brought me the gift of presence. She offered me the wisdom of how being in full-bodied presence and awareness is magnetic. Willow

Imagine asking your wisdom guide about any menstrual symptoms, health challenges, or life circumstances you are struggling with currently and write out their wisdom guidance for you.

Write about any times in your life when you have resembled your wisdom guide in any way. Have you ever supported any friends or loved ones looking or sounding like that? Have you ever approached any circumstances in the way your wisdom guide would?

What qualities of your wisdom guide do you already feel strong with?

I have been recognizing my mortality, and finding strength in that recognition, it gives me the power to take responsibility for my life in a cool and clear-sighted way. What I am learning now is how to do that and not harden up with it, to be active and effective but to stay soft and open and feminine. It is a much slower, heavier kind of energy that takes a bit of concentration to tune in and drop in to.

I am beginning to feel that I have strong leadership qualities, or energy, but that I have been confused by the masculine model of leadership, which doesn't suit me at all, so I have often doubted that I have the capacity to be active and effective in the world. Now as I trust not only my feminine wisdom of knowing and seeing, but also remaining in a feminine mode of action, I feel my strength and capacity rising. Pennifer Moonmama

I feel I am strong on my connection with nature, the voices of nature and working with plant stone and animal beings. Hazel

The enchantress has been showing up especially in embodied movements like goddess flow, womb dance, and vinyasa. She also shows up in all ways that I invite pleasure into my life - anointing, touch, song, chocolate indulgence, bathing, showering, laying in grass, feeling wind against my skin, witnessing the beauty of nature. She captivates me through the colors of flowers, the texture of trees, the sensation of soil, the exquisiteness of fruits, the nutrition of vegetables.

Embodied presence when I choose to be in the now. Noticing and witnessing beauty. Feeling the radiance within my heart. Holding sweetness, softness, and intimacy for myself and beloved. Melting in the presence of my cat. Letting my wildness out. Allowing my creativity through. Co-creating with Earth and sisterhood. Willow

What qualities of your wisdom guide would you like to develop in yourself?

I am beginning to understand that feminine leadership emerges naturally out of being strong and sure enough of the way I live my own life that it creates changes more naturally and easefully than trying to make things happen. I just realized that if I want to hold my power as Enchantress then the place to start is with my everyday choices for myself. So, as at the very beginning, what I want to develop is more connection to the feminine, and the Enchantress has a strength and knowing sureness that supports me to do that. I'm not asking any one's permission anymore, or validation. I know what I know, and I am able to act on it, and still keep a sense of kindness and care of the greater whole, instead of having to be militant and defensive, or devious and secretive. Pennifer Moonmama

I wish to continue to develop my connection with my body, listening to my womb and working in alignment with my what new post-menopausal self needs for nourishment and wellbeing. Hazel

Magnetism and receptivity. I am receptive to creative downloads and guidance and I can feel the magnetism of my womb and heart and there is a space inside of me that feels like I am repulsive. This shows up from the core wounding of feeling unlovable and unwanted and so when I do not receive the validation I seek or the results for a creative project, my first reaction is that I am repulsive. I have slowly been healing this wounding. I would love to move from feeling repulsive and to get closer to feeling magnetic. The more embodied I am - the more magnetic I feel. I also witness how there is a story in my that tells me I have a hard time receiving support. I see the ways that this plays out and so I consciously invite in the experience of receiving and allowing myself to be held, supported, and provided for in any way that my soul needs. Willow

What aspects of your life do you feel your wisdom guide could bring healing and transformation to? How can you become more like them in these situations?

She is the person I wish was with me as guide and mentor in my maiden phase. So she can bring some healing and strength to that part of me which compromised a lot of herself to fit in and appear attractive, all those adolescent concerns and limitations. I can stand behind myself and be confident of my own truth. Pennifer Moonmama

She can help me feel that I am loveable and that I am loved. I can become her by loving myself. By validating myself. By experiencing my own magnetism, beauty, radiance, exquisiteness, wildness, and inner enchantments. The more that I witness the uniqueness of the gifts that I offer, the easier it is for me to feel how when I stand in my full power with love that I am magnetic and receptive. Willow

Describe a specific situation in your life that is challenging you and how you have been approaching it without your soul purpose wisdom guide powers activated. Then describe how you might approach it newly as you fully activate your soul purpose wisdom guide powers.

Please describe your experience with boundaries and ethics in your personal and professional life. What have you learned that feels wise about boundaries and ethics that will support you in fulfilling your soul purpose?

I am strong in holding space and deep listening and in asking open "Clean questions" since that is the foundation for being a Soul based Coach. I have done many non-violent communications workshops and inclusive dialogue techniques throughout my 20 years of work experience with international organizations. I have been married to a Moroccan and we have a four cultures son together, so using multicultural non-judgmental and inclusive language skills is part of my personal and professional life for nearly all my life, also because I lived in many different countries myself. Erika

What really stands out and sets this style of leadership apart to me is the emphasis on sovereignty and empowering the mentee to access her innate gnosis and wisdom. I could sense and feel in these discussions that there is a way to lead and guide that also invites mentees to feel how they too are the own leader of their healing and awakening process.

Another thing that stood out to me was how to recognize when the session starts to become about the mentor rather than the mentee and how that might mean that the guide is trying to resolve unmet needs during the session. I noticed that after I heard that, I was even more intentional in reflecting upon any and all personal shares during a session to see if it was me seeking validation or if it was me truly offering service to the mentee's healing process. I found this a really practical lesson to hone in my mentoring skills and to be even more mindful and masterful about guiding in a way that is co-creative, responsive, and empowering. Willow

Please share how you already implement wise boundaries and ethics in your life and how you would like to grow into this more.

As a Helper not trying to give advice straightaway but listen more and more and ask questions, so that they can activate their own inner wisdom where they already have all the answers inside. Erika

I've been even more intentional in my language. I've been more mindful of recognizing when things are my agenda and opinion vs. offering reflections for the mentee to respond to. I've also recognized how I ask for consent more frequently when I notice that I have an impulse to share intuitive guidance that I'm receiving that can be helpful. I've noticed that I'm more often than not receiving those intuitive impulses and instead of sharing all the information allowing it to lead the session and offering it when it feels ripe and after checking-in to see if that would be of service to the mentee.

Sovereignty is a really big one for me. The more fully I step into leading and co-creating programs in my professional work, the more I see that empowering women to activate sovereignty in all areas of their lives is a major motivating force behind why I do what I do. I am really passionate about supporting women to access inner sovereignty by being connected to the innate intelligence that arises from within, as they are connected to their bodies. I bring this into my life by trying to reflect on instances when I am not in sovereignty and am instead in victim mentality. I try to use those moments as an opportunity to reclaim my power. I point this out to my husband when I recognize it within him and more and more am pointing these moments out to people in my life in a gentle way when the opportunity feels right.

Energetic boundaries are something that (I want to focus on). I've recognized that the more sovereign and aligned I feel, the easier it is for me to attend to my energetic hygiene before and after sessions to help me let go of, integrate and take responsibility for any energies from the sessions that need to be attended to. I realize that before I was aware of this, I used to be like an energetic sponge to other's emotional pain and it was easy for me to feel victim to taking on the suffering of others - now I see the way that mentality disempowered me and take responsibility to attend to my energetic boundaries so that I only take on what my soul knows I'm ready to digest and integrate. This is something that I want to continue to work on.

Willow

How do you feel about your ability to use your voice to express your true essence and purpose?

Write about any times you tend to feel restricted in your vocal expression. Are there any topics you find difficult to discuss even though they are important to you? Are there any people you have difficulty expressing yourself vocally around?

Describe any experiences you have had of being silenced.

Describe any experiences you have had of speaking up despite systems and people that were trying to silence you.

Describe any strategies you have used successfully to speak up in the face of silencing that you feel might be helpful in your process of soul purpose fulfillment.

Imagine that you might have had an ancestor, or perhaps more than one, that was violently silenced. Write out the story of that ancestor. Then add yourself and/or your wisdom guide to the story and show up in a supportive way for that ancestor. Ask that ancestor for any wisdom they might have to offer you about your current circumstances and write out what they tell you.

Imagine that you had one or more ancestors who felt they did not get to fulfill their soul purpose completely and are counting on you to finish up some tasks for them. Imagine these tasks have been added to the mix of your soul purpose. Describe these ancestral assignments that are included in your soul purpose.

Imagine that you have ancestral allies that are supporting you to fulfill your soul purpose. How might they be supporting you? How might you enhance your awareness and appreciation of their support?

Wisdom

What questions do you have for your inner Wise One? In the next pages, write out your own questions and then write out the answers your inner Wise One has to offer.

Grandmother's Wisdom

By Jessica Huckabay

She found herself at the gate

Covered with dark thorn bushes

Thickly woven with cobwebs

Shrouded in silence

She knew this gate

She had locked it tight

Many years ago

Of late, however

She had heard a voice

Crying

A six-year-old voice

Weeping through the night

Why weren't the nurses tending to her?

She followed the sound of that voice

All the way to this gate

The one she had vowed to forget about

Yet now the cries of this forlorn child

Were piercing the spell of silence

She had cast over this place

They pierced the spell of forgetting as well

Those cries were a call to action

She began pulling away the cobwebs and thorny branches

Searching under the rocks at the base of the gate

For the key she knew she had hidden there

The lock creaked and the hinges groaned

But those incessant cries evoked her determination

The gate opened to a garden of dead and rotting things

Everything she ever wanted to forget

Not feel

She had tossed them all over this fence

Into this garden

Where they had festered

Now she had to clear the piles of rotten forgotten things

Toss them out into the light and air

To dry out the slime

Allow it all to compost down to nourishment

To bring this garden back to life

After wrestling with slimy thorny brambles for a time

She discovered she had cleared a path

To an opening to a cave

The crying voice was echoing to her

From the darkness there

Finally, she would meet this child

As her eyes adjusted to the darkness in the cave

She saw a small thin child

In rotting rags

Huddled in the corner

Shivering and weeping

Slowly she placed her hands on the child's back

Their eyes met and she recognized herself

That part of her that had been hurt beyond repair

That part of herself she had to abandon

Lock up

Forget about in order to carry on

She held her there for a long while

They wept together

"I have come back for you.

I am so sorry I had to leave you.

I can hold this hurt you carry now.

Look, my daughter and my granddaughter

And our ancient grandmothers are here to help us hold this pain"

We all begin singing a song

'Like a ship in the harbor

Like a mother and child

Like a light in the darkness

I'll hold you awhile

We'll rock on the water

I'll cradle you deep

And hold you while angels

Sing you to sleep'

We sing the song over and over as she carries this girl

Out into the garden

The piles of discarded forgotten things

Have already begun to decompose more completely

Providing nourishment for life to flourish once more

We work together to clear out the last festering places

And plant seeds of new growth

The sound of our voices singing

Bring warm sunlight into the space

And a spring of clear water bubbles up from the ground

The seeds sprout and quickly leaf out

Blooms and fruits swell

The aroma of life fills our nostrils

The child is no longer weeping but watching in wonder

As she is surrounded with beauty and life once more

Soon she sits up and takes her own adult hand

Together with herself once more

She steps forth into the beauty

Along the pathway of song

Into the realm of love

This poem is a testimony to healing that can happen even for someone like my grandmother who never found it of value to revisit the past in order to heal. She was very much in the camp of denial about how past traumas were still affecting her in the present. As she aged, her coping mechanisms around this no longer worked as she couldn't keep busy anymore. Her body tired out and slowed down. And the physical constrictions of denial and suppression contributed to her dementia symptoms.

In the last few weeks of her life, she was in a home as she was unable to care for herself and her children could not give her the care she needed. She complained about a 6-year-old girl crying through the night at the home. As this was a home for elder dementia patients, there were no 6-year-olds there during the nighttime hours. Except her own inner 6-year-old who had been silenced her whole life, whose cries had never been heard and could no longer be suppressed.

Another aspect of my grandmother's passing is her reunion with my grandfather who passed away over 20 years ago. They had been together for over 40 years when he died and my grandmother spent the following 6 years prioritizing her sleeping hours as she could still be with him when she was dreaming. This next poem is what came through me as I connected with their reunion. Her passing felt very much like his spirit came and guided her to him. And this union in the spirit realm seems to be their ancestral gift and guidance for us, not just their descendants, but all of humanity. May we all remember this intimacy we long for:

Becoming an ancestor

She looks at the back of her hand as she reaches for his glowing fingers

Her own skin barely remembers what it feels like to contain

Muscles, bone, and blood

Only hints and aromas of these densities remain

As her fingers touch his

The memory of physical touch is strong

And satisfied just enough to ease the longing

Of those long years she lived without his body next to her

But it mixes with a new sensation

A mingling of essence

Free of the barriers of skin

Unhindered by the hardness of bone

Her hand merges with his

And the satisfaction of this deeper older longing

Erases all need to pine for anything or anyone ever again

She feels him drawing her close

At first, she expects to feel his embrace

Warm soft lips pressed against her own

A sensation she had dreamed about feeling again for so many years

But now she feels his glowing lips passing right through hers

Right through the roof of her mouth, to the center of her brain

He kisses her there, creating an explosion of bliss and light

Erasing all residue of her prolonged loneliness

Instantly soothing that familiar ache

Flipping it permanently to its exquisite pleasure form

Then he dives down and kisses her heart

And all of the weeping she held back

Behind walls of functionality

Barriers of getting by

Breaks through these now flimsy membranes of smoke

Flooding her whole soul and his with an ocean of liquid love

They both dissolve into this ocean

And undulate to the rhythms of the planets for an eternity together

Always present for the cries of their descendants

Still bound by skin and other membranes

Longing for the touch of infinity

Thirsty for the waves of love they have become

And in joyful rapture they splash into our lives

Crashing through our insistence on suffering

Or stretch out into stillness

For us to rest upon

Floating in soft silver ripples

Smiling upon this illusion of separation

Tickling the liquid inside our membranes

Into remembrance

Through this process of supporting my grandmother's transition into becoming an ancestor, I have discovered that we can bring great healing to ourselves and our families by tending to these passages. And that we can gain great allies in the spirit world by sustaining our relationships with loved ones when they pass. Granted this is an easier process with me and my grandmother because we already had a relatively healthy, close relationship based on love and mutual care. It might require skilled support from Ancestral Healing practitioners to nurture more difficult or abusive relationships towards healthy supportive ancestral relationships. But this experience I had with my grandmother gives me hope that this kind of healing is possible, even with those loved ones who were in resistance to or denial of healing processes while they were alive.

I will also mention that this healing happened for me and my family after many years of ancestral healing practice. I had many conversations with my grandmother before she died about our ancestral lineage, often weaving connections in the stories that she hadn't considered. I have also worked with my mom even more deliberately as she is very engaged with inner healing work and participates in many of my Womb Centered Healing offerings. One of the beauties of the Womb Centered Healing work I do is that I can focus on my own healing process and it radiates back through the womb portal to all of my ancestors, siblings, and descendants. My mother has often confirmed that she was feeling healing energies moving without knowing that I was engaged in some womb healing process myself. I have learned to check in with her whenever I engage in these healing processes so she knows what is going on.

So, these last moments of my grandmother's life were prepared for, welcomed, and tended to. They didn't just happen out of the blue. I had sung the song to her over the phone, the one written out in the first poem above, during the last hours of her life, offering my presence and energetic connection for her passing.

From this experience I have learned that the beauty of these moments becomes available when we slow down and offer our precious attention, our loving energy, our presence. We are enriched when we open to the intimacy of connection, especially when there is pain, difficulty, death. Death can be a beautiful passage. Thank you Nonni for reminding us of this truth.

PART II: Herbal Womb Wellness

In this segment of the book, you will be guided through a series of self-assessment questions and offered various herbal womb wellness practices to inquire of your womb wisdom about implementing. Many of these questions are about the menstrual cycle. If you do not currently have a menstrual cycle that includes bleeding, ask your womb wisdom what you would experience if you did, or perhaps remember what you experienced when you had one in the past, and answer from that perspective.

To start, please write a bit here about what your menstrual cycle may be trying to tell you, or may have told you in the past about your overall health and well being.

Chapter Three: Elemental Womb Wellness Self-Assessment

Please enter your Ayurvedic Dosha constitution and describe any typical imbalances you notice related to this. If you are not sure about your Dosha, you can find a quiz to take here: https://www.mapi.com/doshas/dosha-test/index.html

Please write about any insights you received from this assessment.

Please describe what you know about your astrological birth chart. What are your Sun, Moon, and Rising Signs? And any other planets you know about? What elements do you have a lot of planets in? If you do not know much about your astrology, you can get your chart generated online with a basic interpretation here including which element is most prevalent: https://astro-charts.com/

Please write about any insights from your astrology related to your herbal womb wellness here.

What elements, Earth, Air, Fire, and Water do you feel are most centrally influential in your life, biologically, emotionally, and spiritually? Please describe why.

Describe your relationship to the menstrual cycle, past and present.

Earth/Spring

In this segment we will examine your relationship with the Earth element, exploring signs of how well-nourished you are that your womb space indicates through the various symptoms of your menstrual cycle and/or aspects of your life.

Describe how you track your menstrual cycle. Do you keep a written record of monthly changes in your body, emotions, and spirit? What symptoms do you track? In what other ways do you notice how your feelings and experiences change throughout the cycles of life?

If you have a monthly bleeding cycle, had one in the past, or imagine you had one, does/did/would your whole cycle from your first day of bleeding to the day before you bleed again the next month usually last under 27 days, in the range of 27-31 days, or over 31 days?

If you tend towards under 27 days this might be a sign of nutritional and energetic depletion. Take a deep breath, place your hands on your womb space and ask your womb wisdom how might you nourish yourself physically, emotionally, and spiritually to replenish?

If you tend towards over 31 days, this might be a sign of stagnation in your physical and emotional body. Take a deep breath, place your hands on your womb space and ask your womb wisdom how might you get things moving for yourself?

If your menstrual cycle is, has been, or you imagine it to be irregular, meaning it varies in length from month to month, what stressors have you been experiencing that might be disrupting the regularity of your cycle? Take some deep breaths and place your hands on your belly. Ask your womb wisdom to tell you what feels disruptive in your life and how you might harmonize things for yourself.

Write about your experiences out in nature recently. How connected do you feel to Earth? When was the last time you walked barefoot outside? Sat directly on the ground, leaned into a rock or a tree, or got your hands in the dirt? If you haven't done any of these things in a while, write about how you feel about that and what plan you might implement to remedy this imbalance and reconnect with nature.

Write about your relationship with therapeutic movement practices like walking, hiking, dancing, Tai Chi, Chi Gong, Yoga, etc. How often do you engage in these practices? What does your womb wisdom say about this? Do you need more of this? How might you implement more movement in your life? Or do you need less? Or is it just right?

Write about your relationship with Earth focused meditation practices like grounding, exchanging energy with Earth, Earth based ceremonies, giving your blood to the Earth, etc. What does your womb wisdom have to say about these practices? Do you need more of this in your life? How might you set that up?

How often in the last 6 months have you eaten these stagnation decreasing foods: beets, black pepper, cabbage, garlic, ginger, leeks, peaches, scallions, rosemary, basil, bay leaves, salads? Write out some recipes you might try with these foods if your cycles are more than 31 days.

How often in the last 6 months have you eaten these stagnation increasing foods: alcohol, coffee, fried foods, red meat, sugar? Write out some strategies you might implement to decrease these foods in your diet if you experience cycles longer than 31 days.

How often in the last 6 months have you eaten these Earth nourishing foods: Soups, stews, cooked vegetables especially dark leafy greens, whole grains, eggs, cooked fruits? Write out some recipes you might like to try with these foods if you experience cycles shorter than 27 days.

How often in the last 6 months have you eaten these Earth depleting foods: sugary foods, alcohol, coffee, stimulants, cold foods and beverages? Write out some strategies you might implement to decrease your intake of these foods.

Take a moment to place your hands on your womb space and listen for Womb Guidance about any foods and/or beverages that might be beneficial to include more or less of in your daily dietary intake.

How regular or irregular of a daily routine do you have? Do you go to bed and get up at the same times each day? Do you eat meals at the same times each day? What other activities do you do on a daily basis and how regularly? How do you feel in general about having a regular routine?

Please describe any circumstances that have disrupted any of your daily routines in the last 6 months.

Take a moment to place your hands on your womb space and listen for womb wisdom about which routines might benefit you to cultivate. Write out any response you receive.

Please describe how your relationships support or disrupt your routines. Take a few moments to place your hands on your womb space and listen for Womb Wisdom about steps you might take to improve the mutually supportive quality of your relationships around your healthy routines. Write out what wisdom comes.

Indicate how you nurture your healthy digestion by checking off any of the following conditions/practices your experience and placing an x by the ones you don't:

- You have an efficient metabolism that you feel extracts all of the energy and nourishment from the foods you eat most of the time

- You are hungry at mealtimes and eat to satisfaction, but not to feeling full most of the time

- You have one or more bowel movements per day most of the time

- You are free of digestive distress symptoms most of the time (gas, bloating, hear burn, upset stomach, constipation, diarrhea, nausea, vomiting)

- You have a healthy microbiome and regularly nourish it with fermented foods and pro-biotics

- You are free of emotional eating habits

- You are free of cravings for foods you know are not good for you

- You eat seasonal, organic, unprocessed, local foods most of the time

- You consider herbs to be an essential part of your daily nutrition

Place your hands on your womb space and listen for guidance about how you might implement more of these healthy digestion practices and conditions. Write out the wisdom you receive.

Please check any of the menstrual symptoms you had during your last menstrual cycle or remember having when you were bleeding. These symptoms indicate excess Earth energy also known as Stagnation.

- Brown or black blood

- Large clots

- Brown spotting before or after your bleed

- Cramps at any point in your cycle

- Shooting pain in the uterus

- Constipation

- Breast soreness

- Irritability/mood swings

Take a moment to place your hands on your womb space and listen for womb wisdom about how you might get any stagnant energy moving to alleviate these symptoms. Write out any insights you receive.

Please check off any of the following Stagnation increasing experiences you have had:

- Abdominal surgery/injuries

- Sexual trauma

- Hormonal birth control

Take a moment to place your hands on your womb space and listen for any Womb Wisdom about steps you might take to further your healing process around any of the symptoms and injuries listed above. Write out any insights you receive.

Please check any of the following symptoms you have experienced during your menstrual cycle. These symptoms indicate a deficiency of Earth energy.

- Fresh red spotting before you start bleeding, after you stop bleeding, or at any other time during your cycle

- Heavy bleeding: Filling 4 pads or 3 cups in a day or more

- Bleeding for longer than 4 days in a row

- Two periods per month

- Bleeding for less than 3 days in a cycle

- Light bleeding: filling only one pad or less per day of your bleed or not needing to use pads at all

- Missing periods when not pregnant

- Pink, orange, yellow, clear, or watery menses

- Anemia

- Intense fatigue

Take a moment to place your hands on your womb space and listen for any Womb Wisdom about steps you might take to further your healing process around any of the symptoms listed above. Write out any insights you receive.

Water/Summer

In this segment we will explore your relationship with the element Water and the wisdom your Womb has to share about this.

How often do you practice emotional release practices including breathwork, body movement, and/or vocal expression? How do you feel about these practices? What does your womb wisdom have to say about what you might need around these practices?

How often do you practice ceremonial/therapeutic bathing, either in a bath tub or a natural body of water? How do you feel about these practices? What does your Womb Wisdom have to share about the benefits of these practices and how you might implement them to greater benefit?

How often do you eat these hydrating foods: soups, stews, fresh fruits and vegetables? Write out some recipes you might like to try to include more of these foods in your diet.

How often do you eat these dehydrating foods: salty crunchy snacks, fried foods, dehydrated foods? Write out some strategies you might implement to decrease how much of these foods you eat.

How often do you eat these dampness increasing foods: dairy (except unsweetened yoghurt), sugar, white flour, excess raw fruits and vegetables, cold beverages, ice cream or other frozen foods? Write out some strategies you might implement to decrease the amount of these foods that you eat.

Please describe how much water you drink in a day on average. What is your relationship with drinking enough water? What are some strategies you might implement to ensure you drink enough water each day?

Take a moment to place your hands on your womb space and listen for your Womb Wisdom about how to care for yourself better based on the information gathered above. Describe the insights you receive.

Please describe your relationship to the Parenting/Nurturing archetype in the sense of you yourself stepping into this role, either with your own children, other people's children, other adults, animals, plants, and/or creative projects.

Please check all statements that apply to you.

- You feel well-nourished and supported to nurture all that you are parenting.

- You feel your menstrual cycle is a regenerative process inside of you that nourishes and gives momentum to your creative processes and ability to nurture others.

- You feel that everyone you nurture is also nurturing you by giving back care and kindness.

- You feel that you have ample space, time, resources, and support to care for yourself.

- You felt abundantly supported and nourished during any pregnancies you have experienced, including during the birthing process and for at least 40 days post-partum

- You feel you are overflowing with abundant joyfully fruitful creative energy

- You feel fulfilled and fully expressed in your sexuality

- You feel your sexual energy and expression nourishes you and all you create

Take a few moments to listen to your womb wisdom about any of the above statements that stand out for you in any way and write out any guidance you receive.

Please check any of the following symptoms you have experienced around your menstrual cycle. These symptoms indicate an overabundance and stagnation of Water energy in the body.

- Menses feel thick and sticky

- White, yellow, green, or clumpy vaginal discharge

- Bad smelling vaginal discharge

- Ovarian or any other cysts

- Fibroids

- Acne

- Swelling of the breasts or any other area of the body, ie: ankles, fingers, face

Please check any of the following symptoms you have experienced. These symptoms indicate a deficiency and stagnation of the Water element in the body.

- Dry skin

- Itchy skin

- Chapped lips

- Less than one bowel movement a day

- Vaginal dryness

Take a few moments to place your hands on your womb space and listen for any insights about what the symptoms above might be telling you and any wisdom guidance about how you might bring your Water element back into balance. Write out any insights you receive.

Fire/Autumn

In this segment we will explore how the element of Fire is burning within you. We will also look at the Autumn season in your cycle and your life.

How often do you light a candle, work with fire in a wood stove or camp fire, burn incense, or sunbath? Describe how you feel about these practices and their benefits. Write about any womb wisdom you might receive about how you might benefit more from these practices.

How often do you eat any of the following healthy fire stoking foods: chili, ginger, turmeric, cinnamon, or pepper? Write out any recipes you might feel inclined to make that include more of these foods.

How often do you eat any of the following inflammation causing foods: dairy, wheat, refined sugar, corn, soy? Write out some strategies for lessening your intake of these foods.

How often do you eat any of the following excess heat causing foods: alcohol, excess spicy foods, fried foods, sugar, coffee, stimulants? Write out some strategies around how you might diminish the amounts of these foods you eat.

How often do you eat any of the following fire dampening foods: cold foods, raw foods, sugar? Write out some strategies to lessen the amount of these foods that you eat.

Take a moment to place your hands on your womb space and listen for any insights about any foods or practices listed in the previous set of questions that you might benefit from including more or less of in your life. Describe any insights you receive below.

Please check any of the below statements that describe how you feel about your inner fire.

- I feel passionate and motivated about my purpose in life.

- I am excited to get out of bed each morning and get involved in the activities of the day.

- I feel my fiery emotions like anger are helpful catalysts for change and converting stuck energy into fuel for growth.

- I have healthy practices to process my anger so I don't hurt myself or others with it but instead convert it into useful creative energy.

- I welcome intense emotions and have regular practices that help me to discover the wisdom in all that I feel.

- I love being physically active and have many activities that stoke my inner fires built into my lifestyle

- I have a healthy balance between vigorous activity and replenishing rest in my life so I don't get depleted and burnt out

- I am not afraid to speak my mind when it might upset others but find ways to be diplomatic and kind whenever possible.

- I am willing and able to stand up and be fierce when necessary to care for myself and my loved ones by asserting boundaries to prevent harm

Take a few moments to listen to any Womb Wisdom that is coming up for you around any of these statements above and write about it here:

Please check which of the following excessive fire symptoms you experience or have in the past.

- Hot flashes or nightsweats

- Infections: Bladder/Kidney, Bacterial Vaginosis, Yeast, Herpes

- Heavy purple, or super bright red menses

- HPV

- Cervical dysplasia

- Cancer

- STD's

- Increased irritability at any time during the month

Please check which of these fire deficient symptoms you experience or have had in the past

- Sluggish digestion

- Excessive weight gain

- Undigested food in the stools

- Depression

- Anxiety

- Cold extremities and/or feeling cold all the time

- Inability to feel or anxiety around feeling or expressing anger

Take a moment to place your hands on your womb space and listen for any womb wisdom about the above symptoms and what steps you might take to come into greater balance with the fire element.

Please describe your relationship with your Soul Purpose. Typically, the premenstrual phase of our cycle and the Autumn of our life, or perimenopause have a lot to teach us about our Soul Purpose.   This is the time when we have birthed and nourished our children/creative endeavors for a while and must get back in touch with our unique soul purpose, evaluating how all we have accomplished aligns with it. Our powers of discernment and our ability to let go of what is no longer serving us are essential at this time. How do you feel about this process of evaluation and re-alignment?

Air/Winter

In this segment we will explore how the element of Air moves through you. We will also discuss your relationship with the winter season.

How often do you engage in breathwork practices of some kind: take 3 deep breaths or deliberately let out a deep sigh in the midst of a stressful situation, focusing on the breath during meditation, yoga, or other movement practice? Describe which breathwork practices you engage with regularly or would like to explore more.

How often do you tend to eat wind aggravating foods that give you gas? Describe any recent circumstances in which you felt uncomfortable because of digestive gas. Take a moment to place your hands on your belly and ask which foods are responsible for any uncomfortable gas you have had recently and write about any insights you receive.

How often do you have trouble getting to sleep at night or wake up in the night due to anxiety or worry? How long do you usually stay up when this happens? Describe anything you do that helps you get back to sleep. Take a moment to place your hands on your belly and ask your womb wisdom about any additional practices you might try to release your anxiety and get back to sleep when this happens and describe the insights you receive here.

How often do you find it hard to slow down and rest because you feel you must keep moving? How long has it been since you felt you got to rest as much as you need to? What practices do you do to help yourself slow down when you get into this state? Take a moment to take a deep breath and place your hands on your womb space and ask your womb wisdom about any practices you might try to help yourself slow down and get the rest you need. Write about any insights you receive here.

How often do you eat these Air aggravating foods: coffee, too much chocolate, black or green tea, sugar, artificial sweeteners/colors, dry, salty, crunchy foods? Write out some strategies that might work for you to decrease your intake of these foods if you need to.

How often do you eat these Air soothing foods: Soups, stews, hydrating fruits and vegetables, healthy fats like avocados, nuts, seeds, olive oil, and ghee, mucilaginous foods like flax seeds, chia seeds, okra, nopales, calming herbal teas like chamomile, lavender, catnip, oatstraw, lemonbalm? Write out some recipes you might like to try to include more of these foods in your daily nourishment.

Check any of the statements below that feel true for you:

- I feel a healthy balance between activity and rest in my life

- I feel a strong flow of inspiration that nourishes my soul purpose

- I feel confident and optimistic most of the time about the direction my life is going

- I feel my energies and emotions are flowing in a healthy, joyous dance through life

- I feel nourished by the wisdom of the darkness and the quiet.

- I feel my soul purpose flowing effortless from my being, fully supported by my inner power and spirit allies

- I feel the power of my dreams and visions guiding my every grounded step

Take a moment to breath and listen to your womb wisdom about these statements and write about any of them that stand out to you as something you might like to grow into and/or something you can appreciate that is already true for you.

Check any air aggravated symptoms you experience or have experienced in the past:

- Bloating and gas

- Hyper verbal speech that leaves you feeling agitated

- Trouble falling asleep at night or waking up in the middle of the night and trouble falling back to sleep

- Getting less than 7 hours of sleep at night

- Getting to bed later than 10 pm

- Over-exerting yourself with exercise resulting in pain, inflammation, and/or injury

- Vaginal dryness

- Dry, chapped, itchy, or cracked skin

- Dry, hard bowel movements

- Less than one bowel movement a day

- Frequent feelings of worry and anxiety

- Difficulty slowing down physically and mentally

- Light bleeding, using less than 2 pads or cup changes a day during your period

- Start and stop and start again bleeding during your period

- Bleeding for less than 3 days on your period

- Spotting but your period never comes

- Missing periods without being pregnant or menopausal

- Menstrual cramps

Take a moment to connect with your womb wisdom and write out any insights you receive about how you might bring your relationship with air back into balance by diminishing some of these symptoms.

Please share about your relationship with the season of Winter, both the yearly season and the winter season of your life. How do you feel about the process of Menopause? How do you feel about the signs of aging you might experience in your body? How do you feel about your ripening wisdom? How do you feel about your soul purpose coming to fruition?

Please check which of these self-care activities you regularly implement during your period (or implemented in the past if you no longer menstruate, or implement regularly as a non-menstruator):

- Using only healthy external methods of capturing your blood: organic cotton pads, reusable fabric pads, free bleeding mat

- Bleeding directly on the Earth and/or giving any captured blood back to the Earth

- Eating nourishing soups, porridges, and stews

- Drinking herbal teas

- Taking time to rest

- Taking extra naps

- Getting to bed by 10 pm

- Using a hot water bottle to warm up your womb space

- Abdominal massage

- Keeping the body warm, especially the abdomen and kidney area

- Taking time for self-reflection

- Giving yourself a break from usual activities, duties, and responsibilities

- Enlisting your loved ones to support you in taking time off

Take a moment to connect with your womb wisdom and write about any of these practices that you might like to implement more in your life. Write out some strategies that might help you to do so.

Chapter Four: Herbal Womb Wellness

Ancestral Herbal Womb Wisdom

Write about any herbs and/or spices that are commonly used in cooking and medicine making that you are aware of from your ancestral heritage.

Imagine you could go back in time visit an ancestor who was an herbalist and made medicine for their family and community. Write about where this ancestor lived, what herbs they used, and what treatments they supported people with.

Do some research about what herbs were used medicinally during the time and in the place you imagine this ancestor to have lived and write about what you find.

What herbs and spices do you still have access to and perhaps use today that you imagined or discovered your ancestor may have also used? What do you use it for today? How does that relate to how it may have been used in your ancestor's time?

Take a few moments to breath into your womb space and imagine a root that travels down from your womb space into the earth, intertwining with the root network of the plant realm. Imagine that you can send information about the imbalances you discovered in the previous chapter through your root into this root network and breathe in the intelligence of the plants through your root. Imagine that just the right herbs that will help you balance out your systems reveal themselves to you through this root network connection. Write out the herbs that present themselves to you during this meditation and how they offer to support your womb wellness.

Do some research on the herbs that came to you in the previous meditation and write out what you learn about these herbs from the wisdom of herbalists and scientific research.

Creating your Herbal Womb Wellness Recipes and Plans

Take a few moments to connect with your womb wisdom and write about the imbalances you explored in the previous chapter. Of the elements Earth, Water, Fire, and Air, which do you feel most called to nourish and balance out with herbs for yourself at this time? Why?

Listening to your womb wisdom again, ask about the severity of your imbalances and which kind of professional support it would be wise to seek out for your herbal womb wellness plan. (This is especially important if you are on any pharmaceutical medication that might interact with herbal preparations, if you have multiple and/or complicated health concerns, if you are bleeding more than 5 days a month and filling more than 6 pads or 3 cups a day, or if you are not bleeding anymore when you ought to be.) Check the options listed below that you feel called to connect with:

- Functional Medicine Doctor

- Integrative Medicine Doctor

- Naturopathic Doctor

- Chinese Medicine Doctor/Acupuncturist

- Ayurvedic Doctor

- Herbalist

- Vaginal Steam Facilitator

- Somatic-oriented therapist

- Trauma recovery trained therapist

Do some research about practitioners in your area or who offer online support and write out some notes about your plans to set up appointments with them to enlist their support in your herbal womb wellness plan.

Take a moment to connect with your womb wisdom and inquire about any reasons you might be coming up with about why you don't need to, cannot, or shouldn't enlist the support of the professionals listed in the previous question. Write out any wisdom or insight you receive about how you might address the concerns you have about enlisting professional support on your womb wellness journey.

Looking back on the assessment journaling you did in the previous chapter, describe what kind of nourishment you most need in relation to the elements in order to balance them out in your system. Do you need to increase or decrease the flow and activity of any of the elements in your system? If so, please describe.

Looking back over the ancestral herbal wisdom you received in the previous segment, select the herbs and spices you feel might support you with the elemental balancing you describe in the previous question. Describe here how those herbs and spices might help with this.

Do some research on the energetic and medicinal properties of the herbs you feel drawn to explore (see book suggestions in the resources segment of this book). Write about what you discover in your research and how this information relates to your intuitive feeling about these herbs.

Take a few moments to connect with your womb wisdom and write how you imagine yourself receiving the nourishment and medicine from these herbs. Do you see yourself adding them to your food? Making teas? Tinctures? Oils/balms? Meads or other fermented brews? Bathing and/or steaming?

Do some research about how to make and administer the types of preparations you see yourself using. Write out what you learn from your research.

Write out some recipes based on your research and intuitive knowing combined that you feel to make for yourself.

Write out a plan scheduling when you will make these recipes, how much you will take of each preparation, and how frequently you will take it.

Take these notes to your appointment(s) with your professional support person/people and make any adjustments to your recipes/plans according to their recommendations. Notice the relationship you feel between your womb wisdom and your professional support team. Are you in partnership with them? Or is there any sense of allowing their authority to dominate your wisdom? Do they validate your inner wisdom and co-create a plan with you? Or do they dismiss your wisdom in favor of their expertise?

Take a few moments to connect with your womb wisdom again and reflect on your answers to the previous question about the nature of your relationships with professionals who are supporting you. What wisdom and insight arise for you about how to move towards more partnership-oriented relationships with your health and wellness care providers?

Chapter Five: Research Resources

Ancestral Research:

www.familysearch.com (There are several other genealogy sites but I found this one to offer the most for free) Write about what you discover researching your ancestry on this site.

Energetic Qualities of Herbs

The Energetics of Western Herbs by Peter Holmes

What herbs did you discover in this book to help you with the elemental imbalances indicated in the assessment section of this journal?

Medical Research on Herbal Medicine

Botanical Medicine for Women's Health by Aviva Romm, MD

What did you learn from this book about the herbs you feel called to work with?

Womb Wellness Professionals

Http://www.wombcenteredhealing.com (Home of the Bio-Mystical Womb)

What kind of support do you feel called to ask for from the people and resources found on this site?

Http://www.steamychick.com (Vaginal Steaming)

What did you learn about vaginal steaming on this site? Are there any practitioners listed in the directory that you feel called to connect with and receive support from?

Http://www.parsleyhealth.com (Functional medicine)

Write out any reflections you have about the possibility of receiving holistic medical care as described on this site.

Somatic Trauma Healing

https://directory.traumahealing.org/

Write about the aspects of your womb wellness journey that might be influenced by unresolved trauma and how you might benefit from receiving support with this.

Acknowledgments

I would like to acknowledge the case study participants in the Bio-Mystical Womb Apprenticeship program who so generously offered their writings on the very intimate process of the program to be included in this book. May their journey inspire readers of this book to delve as deeply and gracefully into their journey own womb wellness journey.

I would also like to acknowledge the womb wellness mentors that I have had the privilege to study with: Kami McBride, Steve and Lokita Carter, Pam England and the Birthing from Within (TM) team, Seren and Azra Bertrand, Keli Garza, and Aviva Romm MD.

I would also like to acknowledge my mother, Teresa Todd-Ingram for her miraculous ability to impart a sense of unconditional motherly love to me throughout my life, despite the challenges and limitations she faced.

And I would like to also acknowledge my husband, Geoffrey Huckabay, for his loving, patient, steadfast, and encouraging support for this project.

About the Author

Jessica Huckabay has been writing therapeutically since a family friend gave her a rainbow journal on her 13th birthday. She has devoted her life to holistic health and wellness and writing has always been a central part of her journey. She has been practicing massage therapy, herbalism, and teaching yoga for over 25 years. Now she teaches weekly Writing from the Womb workshops online as well as other womb centered healing practices through her website at www.wombcenteredhealing.com. She lives in Northern California with her husband, many fruit trees, rose bushes, and an extensive herb and vegetable garden.